ANTI-INFLAMMATORY EATING FOR A

Happy, Healthy Brain

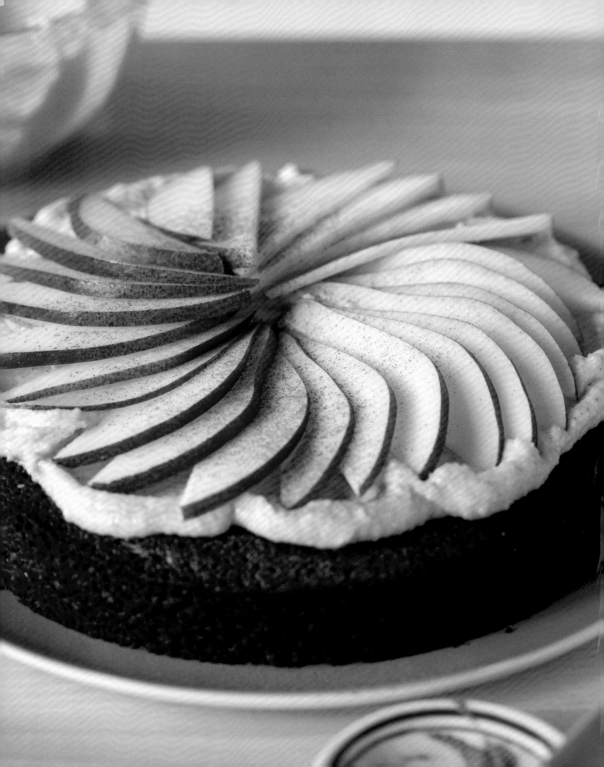

ANTI-INFLAMMATORY EATING FOR A

Happy, Healthy Brain

»»««

75 Recipes for Alleviating Depression, Anxiety, and Memory Loss

MICHELLE BABB, MS, RD, CD
Foreword by Jeffrey Bland, PhD
Photography by Hilary McMullen

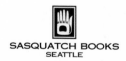

SASQUATCH BOOKS
SEATTLE

This book is dedicated to all of my extraordinary clients, whose desire to eat better inspires me every day and makes me incredibly grateful that I have the privilege to do this work

»»««

Printed in China

Published by Sasquatch Books

20 19 18 17 16   9 8 7 6 5 4 3 2 1

Editor: Gary Luke
Production editor: Emma Reh
Design: Anna Goldstein
Photographs: Hilary McMullen
Food styling: Julie Hopper
Copyeditor: Rachelle Longé McGhee

Library of Congress Cataloging-in-Publication Data is available.

ISBN: 978-1-63217-055-2

Sasquatch Books
1904 Third Avenue, Suite 710
Seattle, WA 98101
(206) 467-4300
www.sasquatchbooks.com
custserv@sasquatchbooks.com

Contents

>»>»«««

Recipe List

»»««

MIND-ALTERING MAIN DISHES

WELL-ADJUSTED ACCOMPANIMENTS

GUT-HARMONIZING HELPERS

TANTALIZING TREATS

Foreword

>> >> << <<

Rubor, calor, dolor, and tumor—redness, heat, pain, and swelling; these were the terms that the Roman scholar Celsus used in the first century AD to describe what we now call *inflammation*. Most of us are very familiar from personal experience with the inflammation that occurs on our skin as a result of an injury or infection. We might also have personal experience with inflammation due to an injury to a joint or part of our body or as a result of arthritic changes. But the impact of inflammation is now seen to be much broader than the traditional view of redness, heat, pain, and swelling. It is now recognized that virtually every chronic disease, including heart disease, diabetes, cancer, and dementia, is associated with a state of systemic inflammation. Systemic inflammation means that it is found within the body and not as easily recognized by the traditional signs of redness and swelling. Heart disease has been found to be associated with inflammation of the heart and arteries. Diabetes is associated with inflammation of the pancreas and body fat. Dementia is associated with inflammation of the brain.

Where does this inflammation come from? Here is where the story gets very interesting and why a cookbook that is focused on producing an anti-inflammatory effect in the body is important. It has been determined that part of the origin of systemic inflammation is the way we eat. Eating too many calories, too much fat and sugar, white flour products, food allergens, food-borne chemicals, and bacterial contamination can all contribute to systemic inflammation and increase the risk of chronic disease. Before this happens, however, systemic inflammation may just make a person feel crummy. People with chronic systemic inflammation complain of symptoms of low energy, fatigue, sleep disturbance, foggy brain, and painful joints and muscles.

This is why the amazing *Anti-Inflammatory Eating for a Happy, Healthy Brain* is so important. Michelle Babb, who is a registered dietitian and has a master's degree in nutrition, is an expert in the use of food in the management of chronic systemic inflammation. Her years of experience in guiding her clients on dietary approaches to regain their health comes through loud and clear in this wonderful book. This is a "how-to" book that also addresses the "why to" in a very understandable and usable structure. This book represents a simple and easy way to implement an anti-inflammation lifestyle using food, nutrition, and diet as the guide. I have been in the field of medical nutrition for more than thirty years, and I find *Anti-Inflammatory Eating for a Happy, Healthy Brain* to be a trusted and well-documented source of information on how to use foods to create a healthy approach to reducing chronic inflammation.

For many readers this book will be very important in finding a path for improving brain health and reducing the risk of cognitive impairment. For others this book will represent a wonderful way to introduce tasty meals and vibrant foods into their lives to reduce the unnecessary burden of inflammation that results in chronic pain and risk of chronic disease. No matter what the specific motivation for reading this book might be, it will deliver an understanding of the relationship between your diet and inflammation and what to do about it that will stick with you for life.

—JEFFREY BLAND, PhD, FACN, FACB, CNS
President, Personalized Lifestyle Medicine Institute
Author of The Disease Delusion
January 2016

Introduction

»»««

There's a TV ad from the '80s that is permanently etched in my mind: A close-up shot of a frying pan with a puddle of sizzling butter, ominous music, and a voice-over that says, "This is drugs." Pause. Then an egg gets cracked into the pan of hissing, bubbling grease, and the voice-over states, "This is your brain on drugs. Any questions?"

Not only is it a memorable antidrug visual, but it's ironically applicable to how food impacts brain function. It's no accident that there's a direct correlation between an increase in consumption of sugar-laden, highly processed, deep-fried foods and a steady rise in depression, anxiety, and mood disorders. In one study involving over one thousand women ages twenty to ninety-three, researchers found a direct correlation between a Western diet and an increase in major depression and dysthymia (chronic depression that lasts two years or longer). The Western diet was defined as a diet comprising processed meats, pizza, burgers, white bread, sugar, flavored milk drinks, and beer.

Nearly all of the commonly consumed foods in the Western diet are known to be pro-inflammatory, particularly meat, white flour, and sugar. Conversely, foods such as fish, fruit, vegetables, and whole grains are associated with less inflammation in the body. Now that we're developing a better understanding of the gut-brain connection and how inflammation plays a definitive role in depression and neurodegenerative disorders, we can start identifying ways to use food to improve and safeguard brain function.

As it turns out, the bacterial environment in your gut, also known as the microbiome, is an important predictor of how the brain functions. Dr. David Perlmutter states in his book *Brain Maker*, "Chronic inflammation and free radical damage are concepts that lie front and center in neuroscience today, but no pharmaceutical approach can come anywhere close to a dietary prescription for managing your intestinal bacteria." I like to think of the microbiome as the ultimate ecosystem of the body. It includes somewhere in the neighborhood of ten thousand species of microbes that cross talk with other cells, organs, and tissues in the body in ways that can be harmonious, neutral, or detrimental. When we neglect or abuse this delicate ecosystem with overuse of processed foods, antibiotics, alcohol, and other prescription and recreational drugs, and add a hefty dose of chronic stress, we set ourselves up for neuro-gastro disaster. The good news is we can choose to support our ecosystem in a way that favors optimal mental health and sustainable wellness.

As a dietitian who works with a large population of patients who suffer from some form of depression, anxiety, and/or cognitive decline, I get inspired by the notion that diet and lifestyle changes can be more effective than drugs in addressing the root cause of these imbalances. My patients feel empowered when they make simple changes in their eating patterns and start to experience mood stability, energy improvement, and clearer focus. This is not to say that prescription medications don't have a time and place, but many of my patients are severely impacted by the common side effects and/or don't wish to have a reliance on any form of medication.*

So what constitutes an anti-inflammatory diet that supports a robust microbiome and a healthy gut-brain connection? All roads lead us back to a Mediterranean-style diet that features a wide variety of plant-based foods, an ample amount of healthy fats, and a selective array of high-quality proteins. Comparative studies show that the prevalence of mental health disorders is lower in Mediterranean countries than in countries that have a more western-ized diet. The true beauty of this way of eating is that the food is exciting and delicious *and* preparation does not have to be overly complicated. Some of the best meals I had in my Mediterranean travels included simply prepared fresh

---

*NOTE: Always consult your prescribing physician for guidance on reducing or weaning off medications. *Do not* abruptly stop taking antidepressant or antianxiety medications without first discussing it with your doctor.

fish and perfectly seasoned vegetables that were just harvested—and a nice glass of wine, of course.

The recipes in this book feature foods and spices that actively help support the gut, regulate the immune system, and tone down inflammation. You'll learn how to get creative with kale, a superfood that's packed with vitamin K, which is a powerful antioxidant that supports the immune system and shuts down inflammation. You'll experiment with turmeric, the featured spice in curry that works in a similar fashion as nonsteroidal anti-inflammatory drugs but without the side effects. And get ready to enjoy the brain-boosting powers of omega-3 fatty acids found in fish with the help of a variety of irresistible fish recipes.

As I was developing these recipes, I took into account the fact that people with depression and anxiety often struggle with a lack of energy, self-motivation, and confidence in their cooking skills. You'll find that many of the ingredients and spices are repeated throughout the book, so once your pantry is stocked it becomes progressively easier to pull together a healthy meal. There's a Difficulty Meter for each recipe indicating how challenging it may be, so you can start with quick and simple preparations and work your way up. I've also made note of shortcuts that you can use to make some of the recipes even easier, so be on the lookout for those helpful hints and make no apologies for taking the path of least resistance.

You'll find a number of other useful tools in this book, including a chart of some of the most powerful brain foods, tips on how to stock your pantry, sample shopping lists and menu plans, and seventy-five recipes that will rock your world. So this is *your* brain on food—good, clean, whole food. It's a happy, healthy, well-nourished brain that functions with ease and efficiency throughout your life. So get cookin'!

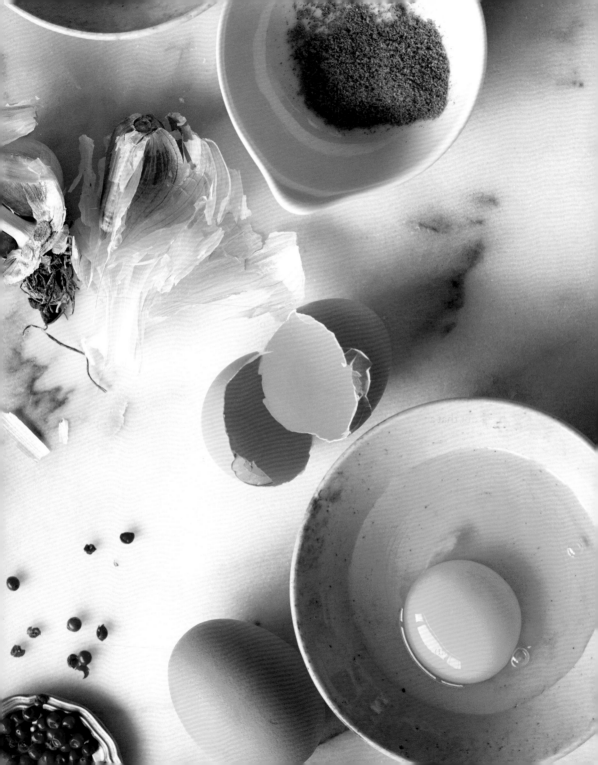

Your Brain on Food

>» »» «« «<

IS THE STANDARD AMERICAN DIET
MAKING US SAD?

There's no question that the Standard American Diet (SAD) tends to be more pro-inflammatory and much lower in antioxidants due to overconsumption of processed foods and a deficit of fresh fruits and vegetables. In one study, researchers discovered an association between oxidative stress and suicide attempts. Those who had attempted suicide had significantly higher levels of oxidative metabolites in their blood as well as lower antioxidant levels.

The obvious question becomes, are there healthier foods or food compounds that can elicit a positive effect on brain chemistry and help combat sadness and depression? One thing we know for certain is that the incidence of depression is much lower in Mediterranean countries compared with the United States. It turns out that adherence to a Mediterranean diet may be one of the most import- ant factors: In a large prospective cohort study involving more than ten thou- sand participants, researchers evaluated the role of the overall Mediterranean diet and individual components of that diet in the development of depression. Results revealed a 30 percent lower risk of clinical depression in subjects who adhered to a Mediterranean diet. There were statistically significant differences in those who consumed more fruits, nuts, legumes, fish, and monounsaturated fats (versus saturated fats). Consumption of meat and full-fat dairy, on the other hand, was associated with higher depression scores.

Another hallmark of the Standard American Diet is a higher-than-average ratio of omega-6 to omega-3 fatty acids. Omega-6 fatty acids are prevalent in soybean, canola, and corn oils, which are commonly used in processed foods. The American diet often has a ratio as high as 17:1. It's expected and appropriate to be consuming more omega-6s than omega-3s simply because there are more abundant food sources of omega-6s, but when that ratio gets weighted too heavily on the omega-6 side, it can lead to trouble. While there has not been complete consensus on the ideal ratio of omega-6 to omega-3, there is some agreement that an optimal ratio would be closer to 4:1. The grossly disproportionate ratio from the Standard American Diet has been associated with inflammation and has also demonstrated a connection with increased incidence of depression.

Couple the imbalance of fatty acids with an alarming amount of sugar that is characteristic of the Standard American Diet and it becomes even more evident why so many of my clients are struggling with depression, anxiety, and general mood disturbances. Sugar consumption has more than doubled since the early 1900s. The average American eats an astonishing 120 to 150 pounds of sugar each year! And we're just now learning of the implications this might have on mental health and chronic disease.

British psychiatric researcher Malcolm Peet noted that diabetes and heart disease occur with increasing frequency in people with schizophrenia and major depression. Numerous studies have shown a link between diet and diabetes and heart disease, but there have been very few studies on the correlation between diet and mental illness. So Peet conducted a cross-cultural analysis that included data from sixteen countries. The study confirmed that numerous dietary constituents appear to worsen the outcome of those with depression and schizophrenia, but high sugar consumption was the predominant predictor of worsening symptoms.

Sugar suppresses the activity of a key hormone in the brain called brain-derived neurotrophic factor (BDNF), which triggers the formation of new neuronal connections and is markedly low in people with depression and schizophrenia. An animal study revealed that a mere two months on a high-fructose corn syrup diet significantly reduced BDNF and negatively impacted learning and behavior.

FROM FAST FOOD TO FOCUSED EATING

Meet "Anna," a forty-two-year-old single mother who works full-time as a nurse. When she came to see me, she was struggling with severe fatigue, depression, anxiety, and difficulty with short-term memory. Although she had taken medications for depression and anxiety at different points in her life, she experienced some undesirable side effects and was looking for a way to improve her energy and stabilize her mood in a more natural way.

Anna admitted to having a "less than perfect" diet and was apologetic about her lack of motivation to cook and her heavy reliance on processed and fast food. She was guilt ridden about feeding her thirteen-year-old son processed foods and cruising through the drive-through when schedules got crazy. Her son was becoming self-conscious about his weight and was also suffering from ADHD. As with many busy parents, this mom was desperate to do better for her child and hopeful that she could improve her own health.

At the first visit, we agreed that Anna and her son would start the day with a smoothie (they both skipped breakfast most of the time), and she would make a slow-cooker meal on a day off so there would be leftovers for at least two dinner meals.

TWO-WEEK FOLLOW-UP: Anna reported that she and her son were having smoothies every morning, eating dinner at home more frequently, and had not been through the fast-food drive-through for over a week. She noted a slight improvement in energy but was still feeling fatigued with low moods and occasional anxiety. Anna was accustomed to starting her day with coffee and often drank up to four mugs of coffee per day and a large soda in the afternoon. Anna agreed to drink her smoothie before coffee in the morning and replace the afternoon soda with a small snack of an apple and nuts plus green tea, herbal tea, or water.

FOUR-WEEK FOLLOW-UP: Anna was surprised to note that drinking coffee after breakfast resulted in an overall decrease in coffee consumption. And while she still craved soda occasionally, she was enjoying a new afternoon routine that included a healthy snack and some herbal tea. Anna reported a noticeable decrease in anxiety and less afternoon fatigue. She was eager to build on her nutrition plan and agreed to establish a day once a week to spend a few hours doing some basic meal planning and grocery shopping. She and her son would work together to wash and chop veggies, make a salad, and make one simple recipe for leftovers (e.g., soup, stew, or chili).

CONTINUED

SIX-WEEK FOLLOW-UP: While still working on refining her food prep routine, Anna happily admitted that both she and her son were eating much better. They hadn't been through a drive-through in weeks, and the refrigerator was stocked with healthy foods that were ready to eat. "I can't tell you how gratifying it is to see my son open the refrigerator and pull out some chopped veggies and hummus for a snack!" Anna was noticing that her own moods felt more stable and reported that her son seemed to have better focus to complete his homework.

TWELVE-WEEK FOLLOW-UP: Three months after our first session, Anna was feeling confident about some of the habits she and her son were forming. The breakfast smoothies were still part of their daily routine, and food prep (while still less consistent) was proving to be crucial to sustaining healthy eating through the week. Anna recounted one episode of feeling overwhelmed and having a fast-food meal that she and her son ate in the car while racing to their next commitment. She noted that they both felt horrible, and she described it as a "food hangover" that seemed to last for a couple days. After that experience, she was even more committed to staying true to her lifestyle changes.

THE INFLAMED BRAIN

When I'm teaching anti-inflammatory cooking classes, I open the class by asking what people think of when they hear the word *inflammation*. The responses I hear most often are pain, arthritis, and joint aches. It's true that these are some of the more obvious symptoms of inflammation. But now that we can measure inflammatory markers in the blood, we see undeniable connections with an array of other conditions—many of which relate to mood and memory. Most people might not think of this as classic inflammation because it doesn't really manifest as physical pain but rather as emotional or psychological pain.

Inflammation is an adaptive process that happens in response to injury. When you get hurt, your body acts quickly to recruit white blood cells and other healing helpers to the site of the injury so repair and recovery can occur.

That's a very normal process, and once the injury is repaired the inflammatory signals are extinguished and the body returns to a happy, homeodynamic state . . . unless it doesn't. When we're dealing with a myriad of factors that are constantly triggering the inflammatory alarm system, those signals become maladaptive and the body gets confused and sick. A few factors that contribute to chronic inflammation include:

» Standard American Diet—highly processed and devoid of vegetables
» Sugar overload
» Food and environmental allergies
» Digestive disorders
» Autoimmune conditions
» Medications/drugs
» Stress
» Lack of sleep
» Environmental toxins
» Obesity (fat tissue produces its very own inflammatory signals)

THE GUT-BRAIN CONNECTION

Allergies or sensitivities to certain foods can cause numerous physical symptoms, including digestive distress, congestion, rashes, hives, and even anaphylaxis. But can these food sensitivities influence mood and behavior? Research is limited in this area, but emerging science on the gut-brain connection provides compelling evidence that the environment in our gut has a much larger impact on neurological function than we ever imagined and that the microbiota in the gut is actively participating in gut-brain communication.

The field of neurogastroenterology emerged from the desire to better understand the fascinating cross talk between the autonomic nervous system (ANS) in the brain and the enteric nervous system (ENS) in the gut. The ENS has been deemed "the second brain," and this brain in our gut may hold the key to understanding some chronic conditions that are not easily explained by the current medical model.

There are between two hundred and six hundred million neurons in the gut that communicate bidirectionally with the brain. This might explain why diagnoses of anxiety and depression are seen in up to 60 percent of patients with gastrointestinal disorders such as irritable bowel syndrome (IBS). Brain imaging in IBS patients actually shows greater activation of regions in the brain that are associated with emotional arousal.

Gut-to-brain signaling is also what creates positive and negative feelings that become associated with certain food experiences in infancy and childhood and may lay the foundation for eating behaviors in adulthood. Clients commonly describe food aversions that emerged early in life as a result of a negative physiological experience, such as severe abdominal pain and bloating induced by drinking milk. Or development of a strong affinity for foods that became associated with reward as a child, like cookies or pastries. Brain imaging in obese individuals shows enhanced activity in the reward center of the brain when viewing images of tasty treats in anticipation of eating them. Sadly, when they actually eat the foods, there is less of an activation of the reward center of the brain, causing the desire for more, *more*, MORE! As is the case with many compulsive overeaters, the anticipation of "food as reward" is mismatched with the actual experience of eating the food and the emotional state that follows.

HELLO, MY NAME IS MARY AND I'M A SUGAR ADDICT

One of my favorite ways to work with people is to facilitate small groups of ten to fifteen people who come together once a week to encourage and motivate each other to make lifestyle changes. I use my training from the Center for Mind-Body Medicine to lead the group through exercises that give them awareness of some of their obstacles and provide them with tools to break patterns that are no longer serving them.

One of the more popular groups I lead is called the Sugar Busters Group. In the first meeting, when I ask participants what drew them to the group, they all mention a powerful addiction to sugar and scold themselves for not having the willpower to leave the candy in the bowl or walk past the tray of cookies in the break room. When I describe the physiological addiction to sugar and note that it actually causes a dopamine release in the brain, I start to see a glimmer of relief on the faces in the group. I compare it to other addictions, like alcohol or drugs, and point out that we would never have the expectation that an addict could refuse his/her drug of choice if it was in plain sight and within reach all day long. The group participants begin to nod and recognize that they are, in very similar ways, powerless to their sugar addiction.

In that first meeting I provide information about a modified elimination diet, which emphasizes anti-inflammatory, Mediterranean-style eating and eliminates sugar, alcohol, wheat, and dairy. I ask the group to read labels and avoid all sucrose, evaporated cane juice, high-fructose corn syrup, and artificial sweeteners. They're encouraged to rely on fruit to squelch their sugar cravings and to eat a balanced meal or snack that includes protein every three to four hours throughout the day. When they eliminate wheat, dairy, and sugar, it rules out 90 percent of the addictive junk foods that are serving as "the drug." The focus is on colorful, whole foods that are mini-mally processed. They follow these guidelines for three to four weeks, and then we discuss transition.

One of the women in the group (we'll call her "Mary") came into that first meeting feeling depressed and defeated. "I binge on sugar every single day, and I'm not sure I can give it up," she said with tears in her eyes. "I know I reward myself with chocolate, but then it just feels like the chocolate takes over and I lose myself completely." I encouraged her to use a strategy that's common in Alcoholics Anonymous or Overeaters Anonymous, which is to

CONTINUED

concentrate on getting through the day without sugar moment by moment. Not to worry about making a lifelong commitment to never eat sugar again, but to focus on providing her body with nourishing foods at regular intervals, minimizing exposure to trigger foods, and being present and intentional in every choice.

Mary came back the next week and was elated to report that she had completely avoided sugar all week. "The first few days were the hardest," she said. "But I'm already starting to notice less of a craving and I just feel more steady and grounded overall."

Mary came back week after week with the same report. She was not feeling deprived because she was paying attention to eating in a way that was restoring balance to her body without triggering the physiological addiction that was induced by sugar. By the sixth week of the program, she was feeling confident that she could continue to avoid refined sugar and focus her attention on mindful, intuitive eating. Not only was she feeling motivated and empowered by her ability to make intentional choices about food, but she had lost seven pounds and was sleeping better than she had been in years.

MANAGING YOUR MICROBIOME

While it may be uncomfortable to think about the body as host to trillions of microbes, it definitely behooves us all to work on cultivating a more symbiotic relationship with these organisms. In other words, make friends with your bacteria.

If your microbiome has been under siege from overuse of antibiotics, immune system dysfunction, drug and alcohol intake, a poor diet, and excessive stress, it's high time to turn things around. You can reduce the population of those pesky Firmicutes (bad bacteria) and ramp up the army of helpful Bacteroidetes (good bacteria) by eating more probiotic-rich foods that are fermented or cultured (think sauerkraut and yogurt). You can even feed the probiotics with prebiotic foods like bananas, onions, sunchokes, and jicama. It's like creating a selective smorgasbord to make your gut flora flourish!

When the gut is happy, the brain is happy. Preliminary placebo-controlled human studies have shown that probiotics can decrease anxiety, diminish perceptions of stress, and improve mental outlook. In a comprehensive literature review researchers cite a study that showed distinct improvements in mood scores in depressed individuals who were drinking a fermented beverage that included a *Lactobacillus* probiotic strain. They also highlight a French study that revealed significant improvements in day-to-day depression, anger, and anxiety, as well as lower levels of the stress hormone cortisol in adults taking a daily probiotic supplement containing *Bifidobacteria* and *Lactobacillus*. These two strains of beneficial bacteria have been associated with positive mental health. *Bifidobacteria* guards against premature cell aging and improves neurotransmitter communication. *Lactobacillus* has been associated with improvements in depression and anxiety scores in clinical trials.

Bifidobacteria and *Lactobacillus* are strains that are common in probiotic supplements and cultured dairy, but there's a growing interest in how to get more of this beneficial bacteria through food. It's no wonder there's a resurgence of the fermented food movement, with dozens of creative combinations of fermented vegetables showing up in the refrigerated sections of the supermarket. Remember when you could find only shelf-stable sauerkraut, pickled with vinegar and assuredly featuring no surviving organisms? Now you can choose from curried kraut, spicy kimchi, or tangy carrots. These designer fermented foods can be an expensive habit, but making your own is cheap and easy. It just requires a sense of adventure, some faith in microbiology, and a little bit of patience. You'll find some basic instructions and recipes on page 139.

A NOTE ON SIBO

Small Intestinal Bacterial Overgrowth (SIBO) is a condition that impairs digestion and can cause a myriad of unpleasant symptoms including severe abdominal bloating, pain, constipation or diarrhea, nausea, and fatigue. As the name suggests, SIBO is the overpopulation of "bad bacteria" in the small intestine, where it doesn't belong. It can be the result of a severe digestive insult, like food-borne illness, or it can be the by-product of long-term use of antibiotics, gut-eroding medications, chronic inflammation, and/or food intolerances and compromised immune function.

When I have patients who follow the anti-inflammatory diet and eat lots of high-fiber foods—plenty of veggies, legumes, fruits, and whole grains—but their bloating and digestion worsen, I sometimes suspect SIBO or some other digestive dysfunction. When this is the case, I recommend further testing with their naturopath or general practitioner, which may involve a breath test for SIBO or a more comprehensive digestive stool analysis to identify bacterial overgrowth and other pathogens.

FEEDING YOUR NEUROTRANSMITTERS

There are over fifty different substances in the body that can act as neurotransmitters—including peptides, nitric oxide, and cytokines—and all are influenced by the nutrients taken in through diet. The neurotransmitters that have been given the most attention for mood, memory, attention, and sleep include the catecholamines (epinephrine, norepinephrine, dopamine, and serotonin), the amino acid neurotransmitters (GABA and glutamate), and the amine neurotransmitter (acetylcholine).

A whole host of vitamins, minerals, and amino acids are required for the biosynthesis and healthy function of the neurotransmitters that influence mood, memory, and cognition. Deficiencies or dietary inadequacies can contribute to imbalances that manifest in ways that significantly impact quality of life and psychological well-being. What follows are some of the key functions of the dietary nutrients that have the most influence on neurotransmitter balance, and the chart on page 12 highlights food sources of these important nutrients.

- » **VITAMIN B$_6$:** Required for biosynthesis of dopamine, norepinephrine, serotonin, and GABA.

- » **VITAMIN B$_{12}$:** Cofactor in serotonin synthesis.

- » **FOLATE:** Increases dopamine production and acts as a cofactor in serotonin synthesis.

- » **VITAMIN C:** Required for the biosynthesis of norepinephrine and protects against oxidation of lipids and proteins in the brain.

- » **IRON:** Coenzyme in the biosynthesis of numerous neurotransmitters.

- » **ZINC:** Required for GABA biosynthesis and blocks reuptake of dopamine.

- » **MAGNESIUM:** Reduces excitatory postsynaptic receptor activity.

- » **SELENIUM:** Important brain antioxidant that is required in the biosynthesis of glutathione peroxidase.

- » **CHOLINE:** Required for the production of acetylcholine, which is associated with memory and cognition.

MIND-ALTERING FOODS

	Dopamine **CONTENT**	Serotonin **HAPPY**	GABA **CALM**	Acetylcholine **FOCUSED**	Norepinephrine **ALERT**
Function	Plays a key role in pleasure, reward, motivation, learning, working memory, and cognition. Dopamine is made from tyrosine.	Regulates mood, emotion, sleep, and appetite. Serotonin is made from tryptophan.	Produces a calm, relaxed state.	Facilitates communication between neurons and is critical for cognitive processing, memory, arousal, and attention.	Critical for alertness, concentration, and energy. Norepinephrine is made from dopamine.
Food Boosters	almonds asparagus avocados beans beef* broccoli cashews chicken* fish lamb* lentils quinoa shrimp spinach walnuts	almonds asparagus avocados beans beef* broccoli dark chocolate** halibut kale lamb* nutritional yeast pumpkin seeds raspberries salmon sardines soybeans spinach sunflower seeds tuna turkey walnuts yams yogurt	avocados beef* cashews kale lamb* lentils quinoa salmon sunflower seeds tuna turkey walnuts yams	chicken collard greens eggs shrimp turkey	bell peppers brussels sprouts kale papaya raspberries strawberries

*All forms of meat should be from animals eating their native diets; look for 100 percent grass-fed beef, bison, and lamb, and organic, free-range chicken.

**At least 70 percent cocoa.

Dopamine **CONTENT**	Serotonin **HAPPY**	GABA **CALM**	Acetylcholine **FOCUSED**	Norepinephrine **ALERT**
Asparagus & Sun-Dried Tomato Frittata	Powerhouse Porridge	Green Soup To Go	Breakfast Salad Sunny-Side Up	Rise & Shine Smoothies
Quinoa Flapjacks	Tofu Breakfast Scramble	Yam & Brussels Sprout Hash	Kimchi Fried Rice	Salmon & Kale with Creamy Coconut Sauce
Honey-Glazed Walnuts	Yam & Brussels Sprout Hash	Quinoa Flapjacks	Green Eggs & Yams	Lamb-Stuffed Red Peppers
Avocado Boats with Shrimp Aboard	Almond-Coconut Bites	Honey-Glazed Walnuts	Avocado Boats with Shrimp Aboard	Braised Kale
Edamame Guacamole with Crudités	Spicy Tahini Tofu Bites	Avocado Boats with Shrimp Aboard	Truffled Eggs	Blue-Raspberry Kefir
Poached Halibut with Pistachio Pesto	Smoked Salmon Roll Ups	Smoked Salmon Roll Ups	Curried Shrimp Kebabs with Spring Slaw	Raspberry Yogurt Swirl
Sweet & Spicy Chicken Chili	Poached Halibut with Pistachio Pesto	Salmon & Kale with Creamy Coconut Sauce	Slow-Cooked Chicken & White Bean Stew with Rainbow Quinoa	Raspberry Chia Pudding
Lamb-Stuffed Red Peppers	Seafood & White Bean Cassoulet	Slow-Cooked Beef, Broccoli & Mushroom Stew	Sweet & Spicy Chicken Chili	
Slow-Cooked Beef, Broccoli & Mushroom Stew	Zoodles Marinara with Turkey Meatballs	Slow-Cooked Lentil & Quinoa Stew	Zoodles Marinara with Turkey Meatballs	
Delicata Squash with Quinoa-Pecan Stuffing	Mock Moussaka	Crispy Broccoli & Cauliflower		
Slow-Cooked Lentil & Quinoa Stew	Beans, Greens & Grains Bowls	Smoky Yam & Kale Salad		
Beans, Greens & Grains Bowls	Smoky Yam & Kale Salad	Pumpkin-Coconut Custard with Walnut-Date Crumble		
Crispy Broccoli & Cauliflower	Calm, Cool Basil-Avocado Soup			
Spinach-Arugula Salad	Creamy Broccoli Soup			
Moroccan Chickpea Salad	Braised Kale			
	Raspberry Chia Pudding			

(Featured Recipes)

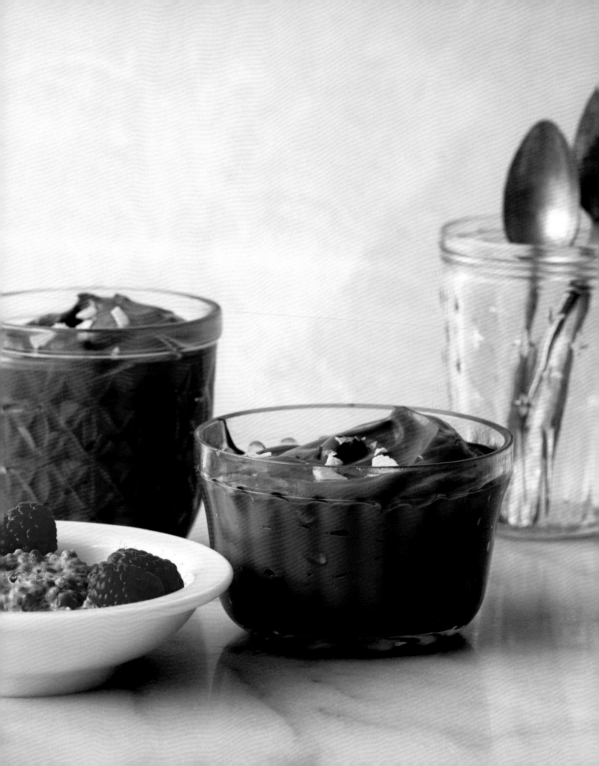

Getting Started—How to Use This Book

»»««

Whether you're suffering from depression, anxiety, and fatigue or you're just looking for simple ways to make anti-inflammatory eating sustainable for you, this book has been designed with ease in mind. Take some time to read through the sections that precede the recipes so that you can start creating a food culture in your home that will support your long-term wellness goals. And you don't have to do it all at once. I encourage my clients to ask themselves what barriers they've experienced in preparing foods that are nourishing. Sometimes it's as simple as "my kitchen is a disaster and I don't have space for food prep." If that's the case, step one is to work on clearing out the clutter, purging the pantry of junk food, getting rid of old appliances, and making space for nourishing foods and useful tools.

You can use the anti-inflammatory pantry suggestions as you start to phase out the old and bring in the new. Once you stock up on some of these staples, the recipes in this book will be even easier to follow and your shopping list will shrink significantly. You'll also have ingredients on hand to assemble quick meals that don't even require a recipe.

The menu plans and shopping lists are organized by foods that can address some of the symptoms you're experiencing. You can be selective about which menu you choose, work your way through all three, or mix and match. If you'd like to do your own menu planning, there are some excellent apps that automatically generate shopping lists based on your weekly meal plan. A few of my favorites are Pepperplate, Cook Smarts, and Plan to Eat.

Once you get to the recipes themselves, remember that the difficulty meter gives you some indication of how much effort is required. If you're suffering from fatigue and low motivation, start with the low and medium-low recipes. As you eat better and your energy starts to improve, you'll be able to graduate to more complex recipes.

Most importantly, be kind and patient with yourself. Nourishing yourself with love and intention is the ultimate form of self-care, but it takes practice. Many of us are accustomed to putting the needs of everyone else first and not leaving enough juice in the tank to take care of our own basic needs—like eating! Just remember that you need to put your oxygen mask on first. If you nourish yourself well and restore balance in your body, you'll have even more to give and you'll lead by example.

BASIC TENETS OF ANTI-INFLAMMATORY EATING FOR BRAIN HEALTH

1. Clean, colorful plant-based foods are the name of the game.

There's no denying that fruits and vegetables are loaded with vitamins, minerals, and phytonutrients that support the immune system and actively cool down inflammation in the body. Not a day goes by that I don't give the advice to eat more vegetables. The foundation of an anti-inflammatory diet is fruits and vegetables. In fact 50 to 60 percent of your plate should be loaded up with these colorful plant-based foods. And the more color and variety, the better. Eating mostly organic produce is recommended to avoid exposure to pesticide residues that might disrupt the endocrine system. If it's not practical or financially feasible to eat all organic fruits and vegetables, check out the Environmental Working Group's dirty dozen and clean fifteen produce list for guidance (see sidebar).

2. Fish is the preferred animal source of protein.

Wild-caught finfish is an excellent source of omega-3 fatty acids, which have been shown to reduce inflammatory markers in the blood and are also important for optimal brain function. Meat, pork, and poultry contain arachidonic acid, which is pro-inflammatory, so I recommend treating these sources of animal protein more like condiments in your diet. If you have concerns about the

DIRTY DOZEN PRODUCT LIST	CLEAN FIFTEEN PRODUCE LIST
Apples	Asparagus
Celery	Avocados
Cherry tomatoes	Cabbage
Cucumbers	Cantaloupe
Grapes	Cauliflower
Nectarines	Eggplant
Peaches	Grapefruit
Potatoes	Kiwi
Snap peas	Mangoes
Spinach	Onions
Strawberries	Papayas
Sweet bell peppers	Pineapples
	Sweet corn
+ Hot peppers	Sweet peas (frozen)
+ Kale/collards	Sweet potatoes

Source: Environment Working Group's 2015 Shopper's Guide to Pesticides in Produce

safety and sustainability of fish, Monterey Bay Aquarium puts out a Seafood Watch guide, which is updated biannually. You can download it or use their app to see how your favorite fish ranks.

3. Healthy fats and oils are essential, and balance is important.

If you're still suffering from a hangover from the fat phobia from the '80s, it's time to get over it. In addition to reducing inflammation, healthy fats are essential for optimal brain function, balanced hormone production, and overall cellular wellness. In order to keep your body in a more anti-inflammatory state, it's important to have a healthy balance of omega-6 to omega-3 fatty acids. Omega-6s are found in nuts, seeds, and oils derived from nuts, seeds, and vegetables. Omega-3s are found in fish and in some plant-based foods like flaxseed, walnuts, soy, and brussels sprouts. The typical unbalanced ratio of omega-6s to omega-3s in the Standard American Diet is a result of overconsumption of processed foods and those fried in vegetable oil. Olive oil and olives contain both omega-6s and omega-3s but are primarily a monoun-saturated fat, which also has some anti-inflammatory benefits. Olive oil also contains powerful antioxidants and phytonutrients that may help reduce pain associated with inflammation.

The best sources of healthy fats and oils include:

» Fish and fish oil

» Olives and olive oil

» Flaxseed oil

» Coconut oil

» Avocados

» Nuts and nut butters (walnuts, almonds, pecans, pistachios, etc.)

» Seeds and seed butters (pumpkin, sunflower, sesame, etc.)

4. Cultured and fermented foods keep the gut healthy and happy.

Your gut is host to trillions of microorganisms that communicate with your body and brain in powerful ways that we're only beginning to understand. What we do know is that the balance of friendly and unfriendly bacteria in the gut mightily influences mood, cognition, and mental function. That may be due in part to inflammation resulting from too much of the bad bacteria dominating the gut, or it may be due to a lack of good guys helping to produce neurotransmitters that keep the brain balanced and focused. Most likely is that it's a combination of the two. Eating cultured and fermented food with live and active cultures helps ensure a healthy balance.

5. Refined sugar and processed foods are not your friend.

The documentary *Fed Up* brought to light some of the more disturbing facts about how sugar and processed foods are affecting our health. The massive increase in sugar consumption is associated with higher incidence of obesity, type 2 diabetes, cardiovascular disease, cancer, and depression. Sugar takes a toll on the immune system, fans the flames of inflammation, and creates an insatiable desire to eat more. In fact one animal study showed that sugar was eight times more addictive than cocaine! Sugar appears to initiate a dopamine release in brain, which creates a temporary feeling of contentment, followed by a sometimes desperate need for another hit. Those who suffer from depression are more susceptible to this addiction.

Avoiding refined sugar can be harder than it seems. As stated in *Fed Up*, out of the six hundred thousand items sold in grocery stores today, 80 percent of them contain added sugar. That's right—if you're eating foods out of boxes and packages, the deck is stacked against you. The best way to avoid the sugar trap is to limit consumption of processed foods and fast foods and opt for home-cooked whole foods as close to their natural state as possible.

HEALTHY PLATE: FOOD FOR THOUGHT

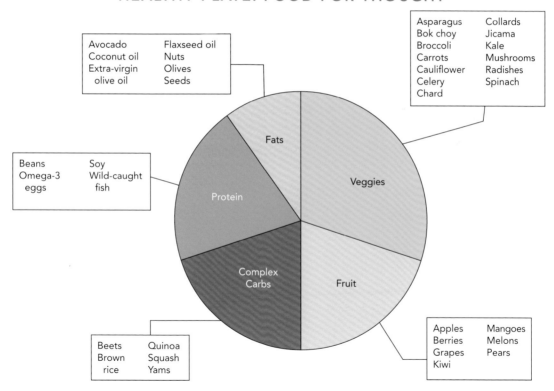

Avocado	Flaxseed oil
Coconut oil	Nuts
Extra-virgin	Olives
olive oil	Seeds

Asparagus	Collards
Bok choy	Jicama
Broccoli	Kale
Carrots	Mushrooms
Cauliflower	Radishes
Celery	Spinach
Chard	

Beans	Soy
Omega-3	Wild-caught
eggs	fish

Fats

Veggies

Protein

Complex Carbs

Fruit

Apples	Mangoes
Berries	Melons
Grapes	Pears
Kiwi	

Beets	Quinoa
Brown	Squash
rice	Yams

What to Avoid

» **REFINED SUGAR:** White and brown sugar (sucrose), evaporated cane juice, corn syrup, high-fructose corn syrup

» **ARTIFICIAL SWEETENERS:** Aspartame, sucralose, saccharin

» **UNRECOGNIZABLE INGREDIENTS:** Read every ingredient list and buy only products that contain ingredients you recognize as food

» **SODA AND ENERGY DRINKS**

What to Limit

» **ALCOHOL:** Limit intake to one drink per day for women and two drinks per day for men; avoid entirely when taking certain medications

» **CAFFEINATED BEVERAGES:** Coffee and tea (black, green, or white) may exacerbate anxiety and disrupt sleep

» **SWEETENERS:** Use coconut palm sugar, agave, Stevia, raw honey, real maple syrup, blackstrap molasses, and real fruit juice in moderation

THE HAPPY, HEALTHY BRAIN FOOD PANTRY

Keeping your pantry and fridge well stocked with foods that support your health and wellness goals is a big step in the right direction. Here are few must-haves:

MUST-HAVES	BENEFITS	USES	STORAGE TIPS
Healthy Fats and Oils			
AVOCADO OIL	Great source of healthy monounsaturated fats; more heat-stable than olive oil	Frying, sautéing, roasting, grilling, dressings, marinades	Pantry
COCONUT OIL	The body uses this cholesterol-free fat as energy	Sautéing, as a replacement for butter or shortening in recipes	Pantry
EXTRA-VIRGIN OLIVE OIL	Excellent source of monounsaturated fats with unique antioxidant polyphenols that have anti-inflammatory properties	Light sautéing, dressings, marinades, finishing dishes	Refrigerator or cool, dark pantry
FLAXSEED OIL	Plant-based source of omega-3s	Dressings, smoothies, finishing dishes (do not heat)	Refrigerator
GRAPESEED OIL	Naturally stable oil that does not oxidize at higher temperatures	Frying, sautéing, roasting, grilling	Pantry
Nuts and Seeds			
ALMONDS	Contain healthy fats that decrease inflammation and help lower cholesterol; rich source of vitamin E	Snacking, salads, topping, almond butter, almond milk	Cool, dark pantry (best stored in an airtight container)

CONTINUED

MUST-HAVES	BENEFITS	USES	STORAGE TIPS
FLAXSEEDS	Excellent plant-based source of omega-3s; unique forms of fiber that improve digestion	Smoothies, topping, egg replacer*	Refrigerator or freezer
PUMPKIN SEEDS	Provide very diverse blend of antioxidants; good source of magnesium, zinc, and iron	Snacking, salads, topping, pumpkin seed butter	Cool, dark pantry (best stored in an airtight container)
WALNUTS	Contain higher amounts of omega-3s than any other nuts, rich in unique anti-inflammatory phytonutrients	Snacking, salads, dips, spreads	Refrigerator or cool, dark pantry (best stored in an airtight container)
Grains and Legumes (all gluten-free)			
BUCKWHEAT (flour or groats)	Very nourishing fruit seed that can be a good alternative for anyone avoiding wheat or gluten	Bean or grain dishes, soups, stews, salads, buckwheat flour	Cool, dark pantry (best stored in airtight container), store flour in freezer
LEGUMES (chickpeas, black, pinto, navy, adzuki, lentils, etc.)	Excellent source of fiber (particularly soluble fiber); valuable plant-based source of protein and essential nutrients	Bean or grain dishes, soups, stews, salads, dips	Cool, dark pantry (best stored in airtight container)
QUINOA	Only grain considered a complete protein, contains small amounts of omega-3s	Bean or grain dishes, soups, stews, salads, quinoa flour	Cool, dark pantry (best stored in an airtight container); store flour in freezer
RICE (brown, red, purple, black)	Excellent source of fiber and antioxidants that protect against type 2 diabetes and heart disease	Bean or grain dishes, soups, stews, salads, rice flour	Cool, dark pantry (best stored in an airtight container); store flour in freezer

*To replace eggs in recipes, combine two tablespoons of ground flaxseed with six tablespoons of hot water. Allow the mixture to set for fifteen minutes before using.

MUST-HAVES	BENEFITS	USES	STORAGE TIPS
Herbs and Spices			
CINNAMON	Inhibits the release of pro-inflammatory messengers in the body; helps regulate blood sugar	Fruit, oatmeal, smoothies, chilis, stews	Pantry
CUMIN	Stimulates digestive enzymes; contains cancer-preventing compounds	Beans, vegetable dishes, chilis, dips, marinades	Pantry
GINGER	Contains anti-inflammatory compounds called gingerols; has immune-boosting properties	Smoothies, dressings, vegetable dishes, desserts, teas	Pantry (dried); fresh ginger can be refrigerated to prolong shelf life
OREGANO	Excellent source of vitamin K, which helps regulate the body's inflammatory processes	Beans, vegetable dishes, chilis, dips, marinades	Pantry
ROSEMARY	Contains compounds that stimulate the immune system, improve circulation, and decrease inflammation	Beans, vegetable dishes, chilis, dips, marinades	Pantry
TURMERIC	Contains curcumin and volatile oils with powerful anti-inflammatory effects	Curry dishes, soups, stews, rice dishes, vegetable dishes, lentils	Pantry (dried); fresh turmeric can be refrigerated to prolong shelf life

A WORD ON SEASONING

There are a variety anti-inflammatory herbs and spices used in the recipes that follow. While I love to experiment with different seasonings, my objective when I cook is always to make the food itself the star of the show. This means that I use herbs and spices as flavor enhancers, but I don't use excessive amounts. If your palate is geared toward spiciness and/or heavily seasoned foods, you might find some of the recipes to be underseasoned. I recommend tasting the dish at various phases of development and adjusting the seasonings to your taste.

You'll also notice that I use a liberal amount of salt in my recipes, which I know some people find concerning. When I get questions about that in my cooking classes, I explain that salt is the ultimate flavor enhancer and good-quality sea salt actually provides some essential minerals. Sodium itself is an essential electrolyte that is critical for cellular function. Some people with hypertension may be salt sensitive, but that's actually fairly rare and many people find they have good results lowering blood pressure just from eating a Mediterranean-style diet, limiting processed foods and fast food, managing stress, and exercising regularly. Needless to say, I'm a believer in using good-quality salt to make healthy, nutritious food even more enjoyable.

TOOLS OF THE TRADE

As you're assessing your kitchen and food prep areas, it's important to think about what types of appliances and tools will make your life easier. Here are a few of my essentials.

Food Processor or Powerful Blender

A good food processor will allow you to blend, puree, chop, shred, and slice with just the push of a button. I honestly don't know what I would do without my food processor, and you'll notice many of the recipes feature it as a tool. I recommend nothing smaller than a fourteen-cup food processor. Cuisinart is one of the more popular options, though more of an investment. There are other brands that do the job just fine, but they run a little louder.

High-powered blenders will often do all of the same things a food processor will do. Vitamix and Blendtec are the Cadillacs of the blending world, and they come with a hefty price tag. Other blenders, such as the Ninja, are plenty powerful and won't break the bank.

Slow Cooker

When energy is waning, there's nothing better than throwing a bunch of ingredients in a slow cooker before you head off to work and having dinner all ready when you walk through the door that evening. There are some fancy models available, but it really just needs a high and low setting to get the job done. I recommend at least a six-quart slow cooker so you can do some large-batch cooking and freeze the leftovers.

Good-Quality Knives

Dull knives are much more dangerous than sharp knives. You'll also reduce your prep time significantly with a nice sharp knife and lots of practice. Wüsthof and Henckels consistently rank well in consumer reports. You can purchase a nine- to eighteen-piece set, but if you're on a budget, just invest in a high-quality, multipurpose chef's knife and a paring knife and then add to your set as you're able.

Durable Cookware

It's time to get rid of your toxic Teflon pans (particularly if they are scratched or nicked). I've reduced my selection of pots and pans considerably. I find that I am perfectly content with large- and medium-size cast-iron skillets. I purchased them at my local hardware store and use them almost exclusively for stovetop cooking. I also like that I can transfer them into the oven. I also recommend a large stockpot along with a medium and small saucepan. One other piece I've recently added to my collection is an enameled cast-iron Dutch oven. It's great for soups, stews, and casseroles and is one of the most versatile pieces of cookware I own.

FOOD PREP FOR SUCCESS

A little planning and preparation go a long way toward creating ease for you through the week. I advise my clients to carve out one hour of prep time once a week right after grocery shopping. For those with a more traditional work week, Saturday or Sunday usually works best for shopping and prep. If you have a less traditional schedule, you might find it easier to do these tasks on a weekday, when there are fewer people in the grocery store. It doesn't matter when you do it; what matters is that you keep it fairly consistent from week to week. I recommend making a recurring "appointment" on your calendar.

The checklist that follows is the one I use when I come home from the grocery store on Sunday morning. I've prioritized it based on what will give you the most bang for your buck, starting with simpler tasks and adding on as you get more efficient with your food prep routine. You can pick and choose and alter this list to suit your needs. If there are other people in your household, think about making this a collaborative effort, and don't be afraid to do some delegating.

The Bare Essentials

☐ Wash all produce (fruit and vegetables).

☐ Chop vegetables for salads and/or snacks.

☐ Store produce in green bags or glass containers (see Storage Tips, opposite page).

Second-Tier Prep

☐ Make a big salad to be used as a side dish or lunch entrée.

☐ Cook quinoa or brown rice (1 cup dry = 3 cups cooked).

☐ Boil half a dozen eggs.

Third-Tier Prep

☐ Make one dish that can be served as a side or a main meal (e.g., Slow-Cooked Lentil and Quinoa Stew, page 102, or one of the Beans, Greens, and Grains Bowls, pages 103–8).

Storage Tips

» Use a salad spinner to dry washed lettuce leaves, wrap them in paper towels, and store in the crisper (no bag necessary). For kale or chard you can just spin it, put the lid on the spinner, and store it in the refrigerator for four to five days.

» Store cut carrots and celery in an airtight container full of water to keep them nice and crisp.

» Store fresh herbs in a small vase or glass that is half full of water (like a little bouquet!).

» Slice wet vegetables (cucumbers, tomatoes) as needed instead of chopping in advance.

» Use green bags to extend the life of your produce. They control the ethylene that fruit and vegetables release, which accelerates ripening and ultimately leads to the early demise of your precious fruits and vegetables.

» Use glass storage containers or mason jars with a half inch of headspace to store leftovers and to freeze individual portions from large-batch recipes.

MENU PLAN #1: ENERGY BOOSTER

Perfect if you are feeling fatigued, lethargic, or overwhelmed.

	MONDAY	TUESDAY	WEDNESDAY
BREAKFAST	Moody Blues Smoothie	Moody Blues Smoothie	Moody Blues Smoothie
SNACK	¼ cup raw pepitas (shelled pumpkin seeds)	¼ cup raw pepitas (shelled pumpkin seeds)	Pear + ¼ cup walnuts
LUNCH	Spinach-Arugula Salad with Curried Pumpkin Seeds	Leftover Mediterranean Pesto Bowl	Leftover Mediterranean Pesto Bowl
SNACK	¼ cup hummus with vegetables	¼ cup hummus with vegetables	¼ cup hummus with vegetables
DINNER	Mediterranean Pesto Bowl + grilled chicken	Salmon and Kale with Creamy Coconut Sauce	Leftover Salmon and Kale with Creamy Coconut Sauce

THURSDAY	FRIDAY	SATURDAY	SUNDAY
Mega-Boost Muesli	Mega-Boost Muesli	Mega-Boost Muesli	Breakfast Salad Sunny-Side Up
6 ounces yogurt + raspberries	6 ounces yogurt + raspberries	Pear + ¼ cup walnuts	We Got the Beet Smoothie
Lentil vegetable soup (such as Amy's brand)	Spinach-Arugula Salad with Curried Pumpkin Seeds	Black bean soup (such as Amy's brand)	Mixed greens with canned tuna and vinaigrette
Smoked Salmon Roll Ups	Smoked Salmon Roll Ups	Hard-boiled egg + snap peas	Hard-boiled egg + snap peas
Tofu Taco Salad	Leftover Tofu Taco Salad	Slow-Cooked Beef, Broccoli, and Mushroom Stew	Leftover Slow-Cooked Beef, Broccoli, and Mushroom Stew

Fresh Produce

1 cup arugula
Assorted vegetables, for snacking
1 avocado
2 bananas
2 cups fresh basil
1 bunch beets, greens attached
1 head broccoli
2 carrots
1 bunch collard greens
1 cup cremini mushrooms
1 English cucumber
1 bunch curly kale (such as red Russian)
1 head garlic
1 knob fresh ginger
1 lemon
1 lime
3 cups mixed berries (otherwise
    use frozen)
4 cups mixed greens, plus more for lunch
2 parsnips
3 pears
1 small head purple cabbage
1 cup raspberries
1 red bell pepper
2 red onions
Snap peas, for snacking
12 cups spinach
1 yellow onion

Fish, Meat, and Poultry

Chicken breasts
1 pound grass-fed beef chuck
1 (4-ounce) package smoked salmon
    (lox-style)

1½ pounds wild-caught salmon
1 can tuna

Beans, Grains, and Flours

1 (15-ounce) can cannellini beans
1 cup red quinoa
¼ cup rice flour
1 cup rolled oats

Nuts, Seeds, and Dried Fruit

3 tablespoons almond butter
¼ cup dried apricots
¼ cup dried tart cherries
1 cup unsweetened coconut flakes
¼ cup ground flaxseeds
6 tablespoons hemp seeds
2 cups raw pepitas (shelled
    pumpkin seeds)
¼ cup pine nuts
1 cup walnuts

Dried Herbs and Spices

1 teaspoon ground black mustard seed
½ teaspoon freshly ground black pepper
⅛ teaspoon ground cayenne
1 teaspoon chili powder
¼ teaspoon ground cinnamon
½ teaspoon ground coriander
1 teaspoon ground cumin
1 teaspoons curry powder
2 teaspoons dried dill
1 teaspoon ground fennel seed

2½ teaspoons granulated garlic
¼ teaspoon ground ginger
2 teaspoons dried oregano
2 tablespoons sea salt
½ teaspoons sweet paprika
2 tablespoons taco seasoning
1 teaspoon ground turmeric

Oils and Vinegars

¾ cup extra-virgin olive oil
¼ cup high-heat oil (e.g., grapeseed,
    sunflower, safflower, or avocado)
1 tablespoon sherry vinegar

Condiments and Sweeteners

2 tablespoons raw honey
¾ cup salsa
1 tablespoon stone-ground mustard
Vinaigrette, for salad

Eggs and Dairy

4 large eggs
2½ cups plain kefir
1½ cups yogurt (plain or Greek)

Pantry Items

3 cups beef bone broth or mushroom broth
1 can black bean soup (such as
    Amy's brand)
1 cup full-fat, unsweetened coconut milk
    (e.g., Aroy-D or Thai Kitchen)
1 can lentil vegetable soup (such as
    Amy's brand)
3 cups unsweetened soy milk
1 (5-ounce) jar oil-packed sun-dried
    tomatoes
1 (15-ounce) package extra-firm tofu
2 tablespoons tomato paste
2 cups vegetable broth

MENU PLAN #2: MOOD STABILIZER

Perfect if you are feeling depressed, anxious, moody, or sleep deprived.

	MONDAY	TUESDAY	WEDNESDAY
BREAKFAST	Asparagus and Sun-Dried Tomato Frittata	Asparagus and Sun-Dried Tomato Frittata	Amped-Up Oats with Mixed Berries
SNACK	Apple + almond or cashew butter	Honey-Glazed Walnuts with Cinnamon Spice	Honey-Glazed Walnuts with Cinnamon Spice
LUNCH	Mixed greens with beans, sunflower seeds, and vinaigrette	Mixed greens with beans, sunflower seeds, and vinaigrette	Leftover Slow-Cooked Lentil and Quinoa Stew
SNACK	Golden Curry Kraut with Beets and Turmeric (or store-bought kraut with turmeric)	Golden Curry Kraut with Beets and Turmeric (or store-bought kraut with turmeric)	Edamame Guacamole with Crudités
DINNER	Rockfish, Mushrooms, and Fennel	Slow-Cooked Lentil and Quinoa Stew	Taco salad bar with greens, beans, chicken, guacamole, and salsa

THURSDAY	FRIDAY	SATURDAY	SUNDAY
Amped-Up Oats with Mixed Berries	Amped-Up Oats with Mixed Berries	Yam and Brussels Sprout Hash with Smoked Salmon	Yam and Brussels Sprout Hash with Smoked Salmon
Apple + almond or cashew butter	Hard-boiled egg	¼ cup raw pepitas (shelled pumpkin seeds) + mandarin orange	¼ cup raw pepitas (shelled pumpkin seeds) + mandarin orange
Leftover taco salad bar	Canned tuna or sardines on a mixed greens salad	Leftover Zoodles Marinara with Turkey Meatballs	Mixed greens salad with Spicy Tahini Tofu Bites
Edamame Guacamole with Crudités	Apple + ¼ cup pistachios	¼ cup tapenade + celery	¼ cup tapenade + celery
Leftover Slow-Cooked Lentil and Quinoa Stew	Zoodles Marinara with Turkey Meatballs	Seafood and White Bean Cassoulet	Leftover Seafood and White Bean Cassoulet

Fresh Produce

3 apples
1 bunch asparagus
Assorted vegetables, for snacking
2 avocados
½ pound brussels sprouts
5 carrots
3 stalks celery, plus more for snacking
1½ pounds cremini or shiitake
　　mushrooms
1 fennel bulb
2 heads garlic
2 garnet yams
1 knob fresh ginger
¼ cup Italian parsley
2 medium leeks
2 lemons
1 lime
2 mandarin oranges
2 cups mixed berries (otherwise
　　use frozen)
4 cups mixed greens
1 tablespoon minced fresh oregano
　　(otherwise use dried)
1 small head savoy cabbage
8 shiitake mushrooms
1 tablespoon fresh thyme leaves or
　　(otherwise use dried)
1 small white onion
3 small yellow onions
3 medium zucchini

Fish, Meat, and Poultry

½ pound bay scallops
1 boneless, skinless chicken breast
1½ pounds rockfish
8 ounces smoked salmon
½ pound wild-caught salmon
½ pound medium shrimp
1 can tuna
1 pound ground turkey

Beans, Grains, and Flours

Beans, for salads
1 (15-ounce) can cannellini beans
¾ cup French green lentils
2¼ cups rolled oats
½ cup quinoa

Nuts, Seeds, and Dried Fruit

½ cup raw slivered almonds
2 tablespoons almond butter
2 tablespoons chia seeds
2 tablespoons hemp seeds
½ cup raw pepitas (shelled
　　pumpkin seeds)
¼ cup pistachios
½ cup raw sunflower seeds
1½ cups raw walnuts

Dried Herbs and Spices

1 bay leaf
1½ teaspoons freshly ground
　　black pepper
⅛ teaspoon ground cayenne
4 teaspoons ground cinnamon
½ teaspoon ground coriander

¼ cup ground cumin

1 tablespoon dried Italian herbs or Herbes de Provence

1 teaspoon ground nutmeg

2 tablespoons dried parsley

1¾ teaspoons crushed red pepper flakes

1 teaspoon dried sage

3 tablespoons sea salt

2 teaspoons sweet paprika

2 teaspoons dried tarragon

4 tablespoons ground turmeric

1½ teaspoons ground white pepper

Oils and Vinegars

Coconut oil, for greasing

½ cup extra-virgin olive oil

1 tablespoon high-heat oil (e.g., grapeseed, sunflower, safflower, or avocado)

Condiments and Sweeteners

1 tablespoon coconut palm sugar or pure maple syrup

¼ cup raw honey

½ cup prepared guacamole

¾ cup salsa

¼ cup tahini

2 tablespoons gluten-free tamari

½ cup tapenade

Vinaigrette, for salad

Frozen Foods

1 cup frozen shelled edamame

Eggs and Dairy

14 large eggs

Pantry Items

¼ cup full-fat, unsweetened coconut milk

1 (16-ounce jar) curry kraut

1½ cups fish stock

1 (18-ounce) jar marinara sauce (no sugar added)

2 cups unsweetened soy milk

1 (5-ounce jar) oil-packed sun-dried tomatoes

1 pound extra-firm tofu

1 (28-ounce) can diced tomatoes

1 (15-ounce) can diced tomatoes

2 tablespoons tomato paste

2½ cups vegetable or mushroom broth

MENU PLAN #3: MEMORY ENHANCER

Perfect if you are feeling unfocused, foggy, or easily distracted.

	MONDAY	TUESDAY	WEDNESDAY
BREAKFAST	Total Recall Smoothie	Total Recall Smoothie	Total Recall Smoothie
SNACK	½ avocado with gomasio*	½ avocado with gomasio*	¼ cup raw pepitas (shelled pumpkin seeds) + snap peas
LUNCH	Moroccan Chickpea Salad	Leftover Moroccan Chickpea Salad	Leftover Moroccan Chickpea Salad
SNACK	Roasted Roots Bathed in Balsamic	Roasted Roots Bathed in Balsamic	Roasted Roots Bathed in Balsamic
DINNER	Whitefish and Broccoli with Lemony Tahini Sauce	Lamb-Stuffed Red Peppers	Leftover Lamb-Stuffed Red Peppers

*Gomasio is a blend of sea salt, sesame seeds, and seaweed.

THURSDAY	FRIDAY	SATURDAY	SUNDAY
Green Eggs and Yams	Green Eggs and Yams	Kimchi Fried Rice	Kimchi Fried Rice
Almond-Coconut Bites	Almond-Coconut Bites	We Got the Beet Smoothie	We Got the Beet Smoothie
Fennel and Spring Onion Salad with Blood Orange Vinaigrette	Fennel and Spring Onion Salad with Blood Orange Vinaigrette	Mixed greens with beans, sunflower seeds, and vinaigrette	Leftover Crispy Broccoli and Cauliflower with Cashew Drizzle
¼ cup hummus + vegetables	¼ cup hummus + vegetables	Apple + 1 tablespoon almond butter	Apple + 1 tablespoon almond butter
Delicata Squash with Quinoa-Pecan Stuffing	Leftover Delicata Squash with Quinoa-Pecan Stuffing	Whitefish Tikka Masala + Crispy Broccoli and Cauliflower with Cashew Drizzle	Leftover Whitefish Tikka Masala + Braised Kale with Roasted Garlic–Tahini Dressing

Fresh Produce

2 apples
Assorted vegetables, for snacking
2 avocados
1½ cups baby kale or spinach
2 blood oranges (otherwise use 1 navel
    orange)
2 heads broccoli
4 carrots
1 head cauliflower
1 pound cremini or button mushrooms
5 crimson beets, greens attached
1 bunch curly kale (such as red Russian)
3 medium delicata squash
1 fennel bulb
2 heads garlic
2 garnet yams
1 knob fresh ginger
¼ cup Italian parsley leaves
1 lemon
2 lime leaves
4 cups mixed greens, plus more for lunch
2 pears
6 red bell peppers
1 large rutabaga
4 shallots
1 cup shiitake mushrooms
Snap peas, for snacking
1 spring or red onion
2 turnips
1 cup stemmed and finely chopped
    Tuscan kale
1 small white or yellow onion

Fish, Meat, and Poultry

1 pound ground lamb
2½ pounds whitefish

Beans, Grains, and Flours

Beans, for salad
3½ cup cooked brown rice
1 (15-ounce) can chickpeas
1 cup quinoa

Nuts, Seeds, and Dried Fruit

2 cups raw almonds
2 tablespoons almond butter
½ cup raw cashews
½ cup unsweetened shredded coconut
7 Medjool dates
½ cup pecans
¼ cup raw pepitas (shelled
    pumpkin seeds)
¼ cup raisins
Sunflower seeds, for salad

Dried Herbs and Spices

1 teaspoon berbere
1 teaspoon freshly ground black pepper
3 tablespoons black sesame seeds
1½ tablespoons ground cinnamon
¼ teaspoon ground coriander
1 tablespoon ground cumin
1 teaspoon garam masala
½ teaspoon granulated garlic
½ teaspoon ground ginger

1 tablespoon gomasio
1 tablespoon dried Italian herbs
5 tablespoons nutritional yeast
1 tablespoon plus 1 teaspoon
   dried oregano
1 teaspoon dried sage
¼ cup sea salt
1½ tablespoons ground turmeric
½ teaspoon ground white pepper

Oils and Vinegars

4 tablespoons balsamic vinegar
2 tablespoons coconut oil
¼ cup high-heat oil (e.g., grapeseed,
   sunflower, safflower, or avocado)
1 cup extra-virgin olive oil
1 tablespoon rice vinegar
2 tablespoons sherry vinegar

Condiments and Sweeteners

3 tablespoons raw honey
½ cup hummus
¾ cup kimchi
Salsa, for Green Eggs and Yams
½ cup tahini

1 tablespoon gluten-free tamari
Vinaigrette, for salad

Frozen Foods

3 cups frozen blueberries
1½ cups frozen cubed butternut squash
½ cup frozen papaya (otherwise use
   ½ ripe pear)
1¾ cups frozen petite peas

Eggs and Dairy

8 large eggs
½ cup plain low-fat Greek yogurt (otherwise use ¼ cup full-fat, unsweetened
   coconut milk
1½ cups unsweetened yogurt or kefir

Pantry Items

3 tablespoons cocoa nibs
½ cup pitted kalamata olives
½ cup mushroom broth
1 (28-ounce) can diced tomatoes
2 cups vegetable broth

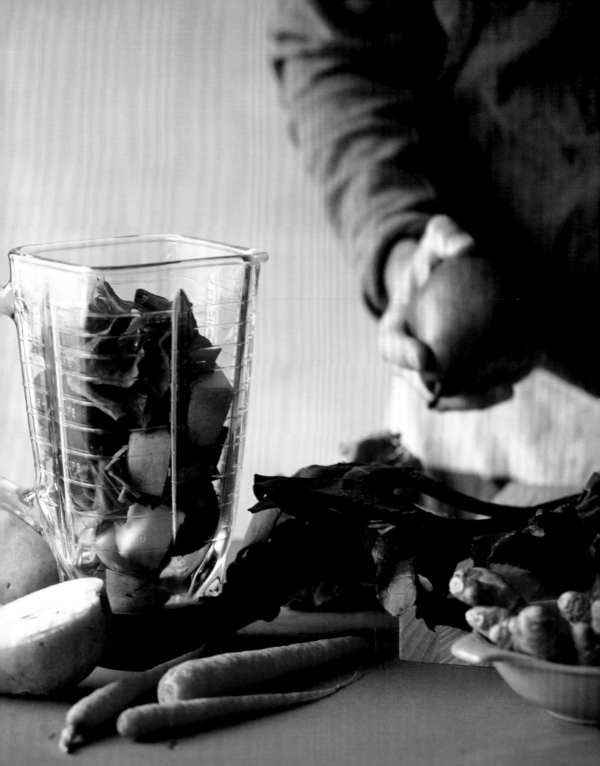

Eye-Openers

»»««

First we eat, then we do everything else.
—M. F. K. FISHER

>>»«<<

>>»«<<

Green Soup To Go

This soup is so simple and would be nourishing any time of the day. I wanted to feature it in the breakfast section because I often find myself reminding clients that eating a creamy soup for breakfast is basically like having a warm smoothie. It's ideal for busy people who just can't find time to sit and savor breakfast. You can simply transfer this soup into a to-go mug and sip on it during your morning commute.

Makes 2 servings

2 cups spinach
1 cup frozen peas, thawed
1 avocado, halved
2 cups vegetable broth
2 teaspoons ground turmeric

1 teaspoon ground cumin
1 teaspoon ground coriander
1 teaspoon sea salt
Freshly ground black pepper
  (optional)

In a food processor or blender, put the spinach and peas. Scoop in the avocado, add the broth, turmeric, cumin, coriander, and salt, and season with pepper to taste. Blend until smooth. Transfer the soup to a small pot over medium heat and warm for 2 to 3 minutes (or microwave in a bowl for 1 minute), or until heated through.

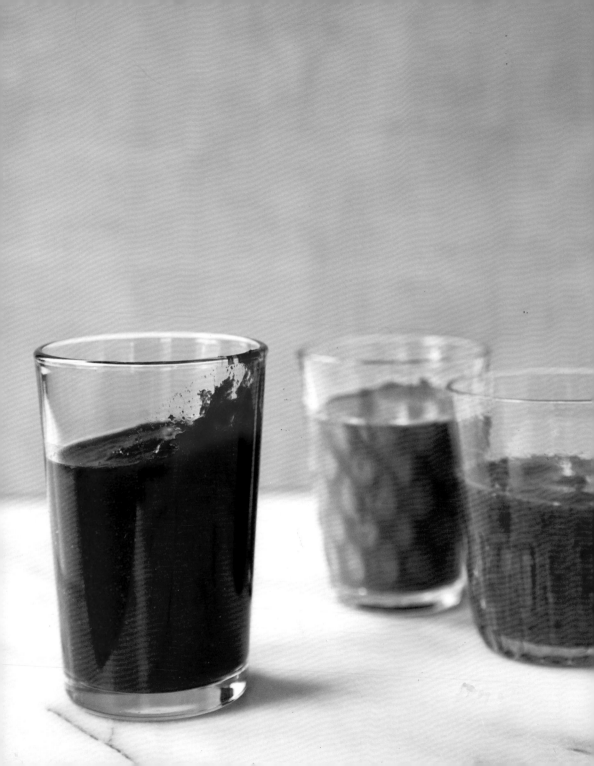

Rise-and-Shine Smoothies

While I'm not a huge advocate of eating on the go, I do understand that morning-averse, busy people often need a quick breakfast they can take with them. Smoothies can be a great way to pack a lot of nutrients into a drinkable meal that can be enjoyed on the road if necessary. They're also often a hit with the kids and beat the heck out of sugary cereal.

Makes 1 serving (each option)

TOTAL RECALL SMOOTHIE (MEMORY BOOSTER)

1 cup frozen blueberries
¾ cup water
½ cup frozen papaya or ½ ripe pear
½ cup chopped broccoli stems
½ cup unsweetened plain yogurt
    or kefir
1 tablespoon raw honey

MOODY BLUES SMOOTHIE (MOOD ENHANCER)

2 cups spinach
1 cup fresh or frozen mixed berries
1 cup unsweetened soy milk
½ ripe banana
2 tablespoons hemp seeds
1 tablespoon almond butter

WE GOT THE BEET SMOOTHIE (ENERGY IMPROVER)

1 cored, unpeeled ripe pear
1 skin-on beet, well scrubbed and
    shredded or chopped
1 cup beet greens
1 carrot, chopped
½ teaspoon minced fresh ginger
1 cup water
½ cup ice cubes (optional)

In a powerful blender, blend all the ingredients for your smoothie of choice until well combined. Pour into a large glass and drink mindfully.

Overnight Porridges

There's nothing better than opening up the refrigerator first thing in the morning and finding a yummy breakfast that's ready to eat. These overnight porridges are loaded with anti-inflammatory, mood-boosting nutrients and they'll hold you over for a few hours. If you don't love eating cold porridge, you can always heat it up. I like to make individual servings in mason jars so my breakfast is already preportioned if I need to take it on the road.

Makes 4 servings (each option)

AMPED-UP OATS WITH MIXED BERRIES

2 cups rolled oats

2 cups unsweetened soy milk (or any milk substitute)

2 cups fresh or frozen mixed berries

½ cup raw slivered almonds

2 tablespoons chia seeds

2 tablespoons hemp seeds

1 tablespoon coconut palm sugar or pure maple syrup (optional)

2 teaspoons ground cinnamon

1 teaspoon ground nutmeg

MEGA-BOOST MUESLI

2 cups plain kefir (see note)

1 cup rolled oats

1 cup unsweetened coconut flakes

½ cup chopped raw walnuts

½ cup raw pepitas (shelled pumpkin seeds)

¼ cup ground flaxseeds

¼ cup dried tart cherries

¼ cup chopped dried apricots

1 tablespoon raw honey (optional)

POWERHOUSE PORRIDGE WITH PUMPKIN AND BUCKWHEAT GROATS

2 cups buckwheat groats, soaked overnight, rinsed, and drained

1 cup canned pumpkin

1 cup plain Greek or coconut yogurt (low-fat or full-fat)

½ cup chopped dried figs (or sliced fresh figs if they're in season!)

2 tablespoons ground flaxseeds

2 tablespoons coconut palm sugar or pure maple syrup (optional)

2 teaspoons ground cinnamon

1 teaspoon minced fresh ginger, or ¼ teaspoon ground

In a large bowl, combine all the ingredients for your porridge of choice, or divide among four mason jars with lids. Cover and refrigerate overnight. The porridge will keep for a week in the refrigerator.

Note: Kefir is traditionally a cultured dairy product, but nondairy forms made from soy and coconut are also available. Kefir is the consistency of drinkable yogurt, and it's loaded with beneficial bacteria that make the gut happy. If you're feeling ambitious, you can purchase kefir grains and make your own kefir using whatever type of milk you like (find a recipe on page 144).

Breakfast Salad Sunny-Side Up

I know what you're thinking . . . salad for breakfast? You've gotta be kidding me! To that I would say, don't knock it till you try it. I love the simplicity of throwing a fistful of greens in a bowl and using the rich, delicious egg yolk as the dressing. When I'm feeling more ambitious, I might put some sautéed vegetables like leeks, mushrooms, and peppers on top of the greens, but most days it's just me, the greens, and two eggs having a wake-up party.

Makes 1 serving

2 cups loosely packed spinach and/or baby kale
1 tablespoon extra-virgin olive oil
¼ teaspoon sea salt
¼ teaspoon freshly ground black pepper
¼ cup water
2 large eggs

In a bowl, toss the greens with the oil, salt, and pepper.

In a small skillet with a lid over high heat, bring the water to a low boil, then reduce the heat to medium. Gently crack each egg into the skillet. Cover and cook the eggs for 3 to 4 minutes, or until the whites are opaque but the yolks are still runny. Use a spatula to transfer the eggs to the greens. Cut the eggs open with your fork to get the full effect of the yolks blending with the oil for a perfect breakfast salad dressing.

BRAIN FOOD FACT

Eggs are one of the best food sources of choline, which helps boost memory and improves cognitive function. As an added bonus, high-choline foods may help decrease anxiety, some studies show.

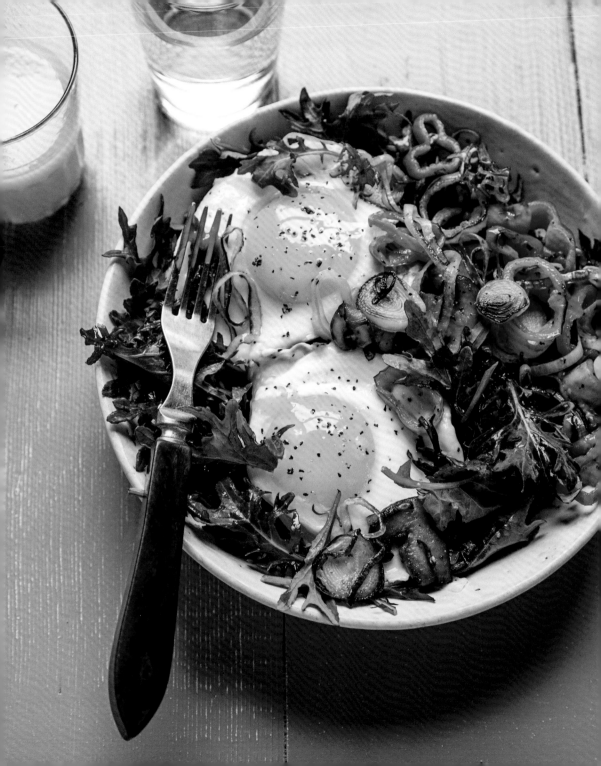

Asparagus and Sun-Dried Tomato Frittata

DIFFICULTY METER
● ● ● ○ ○

The first time I made a frittata I was hosting brunch at my house and was feeling too overwhelmed to do my usual made-to-order omelets. So I gave myself a break and just threw all my favorite ingredients in a skillet, tossed in a dozen eggs, transferred it into the oven, and . . . eureka! Less than thirty minutes later I had this beautifully browned, rustic-looking egg dish that was a huge hit with the brunch crowd. The best discovery was that it reheats well and can be used for a quick heat-and-go breakfast for the next several days. I tell my clients to make this for Sunday breakfast and enjoy the leftovers through the middle of the week.

Makes 8 servings

- 2 tablespoons extra-virgin olive oil
- 1 yellow onion, thinly sliced
- 5 to 6 cremini or shiitake mushrooms, thinly sliced
- 1 cup oil-packed sun-dried tomatoes, drained and chopped
- 1 tablespoon dried Italian herbs or Herbes de Provence
- ½ teaspoon sea salt
- 1 bunch asparagus, trimmed and chopped into 1-inch pieces
- 2 cloves garlic, minced
- 12 large eggs
- ½ teaspoon freshly ground black pepper
- ¼ cup finely chopped Italian parsley
- 1 avocado, sliced

Preheat the oven to 350 degrees F.

Heat the oil in a large ovenproof skillet over medium heat. Add the onion and sauté, stirring occasionally, for 2 to 3 minutes, or until translucent. Add the mushrooms, tomatoes, Italian herbs, and salt, and sauté for another 3 to 4 minutes. Add the asparagus and garlic and sauté, stirring occasionally, for another 3 minutes.

In a large bowl, beat the eggs. Pour them into the skillet over the sautéed vegetables, spreading them evenly in the pan. Sprinkle the pepper over the top. Transfer the skillet to the oven and bake for about 20 minutes, or until a toothpick inserted into the center comes out clean. Sprinkle with the parsley and arrange the avocado slices over the top.

Tofu Breakfast Scramble

Tofu often gets a bad rap because of its unappealing texture and overall lack of personality. But have you ever tried cleverly disguising your tofu as scrambled eggs? Well, this delicious breakfast dish definitely takes on the appearance of a familiar favorite. Crumbling tofu gives it a much better texture and makes it easier to cook to perfection. Tofu is such a great plant-based source of protein, and it contains powerful antioxidants and protective phytonutrients. The addition of turmeric makes this a very anti-inflammatory breakfast. This dish reheats well, so double the batch and have leftovers for several days.

Makes 2 servings

1 tablespoon grapeseed or sunflower oil

8 ounces extra-firm tofu, drained (I like Wildwood organic sprouted tofu)

1 tablespoon nutritional yeast

2 teaspoons ground turmeric

½ cup sliced cremini mushrooms

½ teaspoon sea salt

½ cup chopped Swiss chard, kale, or spinach

2 teaspoons gluten-free tamari

½ avocado, sliced

Heat the oil in a large sauté pan over medium-high heat. Wrap the tofu in a large paper towel and gently squeeze to remove excess water. Crumble the tofu and add it to the pan. Sprinkle with the nutritional yeast and turmeric and sauté for 2 to 3 minutes.

Add the mushrooms and salt and sauté until the mushrooms soften, about 2 minutes. Add the chard and sauté for 1 to 2 minutes. Stir in the tamari, top with avocado slices, and serve.

Green Eggs and Yams

DIFFICULTY METER
● ● ○ ○ ○

This is a whole new twist on the Dr. Seuss classic, and it can be a great way to get the kiddos eating kale for breakfast. You can make this recipe part of your prep routine on the weekend and have a nutritious, balanced breakfast that's ready to heat and eat during the busy week. The egg muffins will keep in the refrigerator for four to five days.

Makes 6 servings

Coconut oil, for greasing
1 garnet yam, peeled and grated
8 large eggs
1½ cups baby kale or spinach
1 tablespoon ground turmeric
2 teaspoons ground cumin

1½ teaspoons sea salt
2 to 3 tablespoons nutritional yeast or
    finely grated Parmesan cheese
1 avocado, sliced
Salsa, for serving (optional)

Preheat the oven to 375 degrees F.

Grease six cups in a standard muffin tin with about ½ teaspoon coconut oil each. Divide the yams into equal portions and arrange in the bottom of each muffin cup. The yams should fill each cup about a quarter of the way full. Transfer the tin to the oven and bake for 10 minutes.

While the yams are cooking, crack the eggs into a blender or food processor. Add the kale, turmeric, cumin, and salt. Pulse several times until the eggs become frothy and the kale is mostly blended in. (Note: I like to have tiny pieces of kale still intact for texture, but if you're making this for picky eaters, you can keep right on blending.)

Remove the muffin tin from the oven and divide the egg mixture evenly among the cups. Sprinkle the nutritional yeast over the top of each egg muffin and bake for another 12 to 15 minutes, or until cooked through.

Serve with the avocado slices and some salsa if you want more of a kick.

Kimchi Fried Rice

One of my favorite summer hangouts is Marination Ma Kai, a casual West Seattle restaurant with an outdoor deck overlooking Puget Sound. This is where I discovered the magic of kimchi fried rice. They top it with a sunny-side up egg, and every time I order it during happy hour I think, "This would be an incredible breakfast!" Play around with the protein options to give yourself different variations on this simple, savory dish.

Makes 4 servings

1 tablespoon coconut oil
1 shallot, chopped
6 cremini or button mushrooms, chopped
2 cloves garlic, crushed
1 teaspoon sea salt
1 cup frozen petite peas
1½ cups cooked brown rice (leftover works great!)

¾ cup kimchi
1 of the following protein sources:
    8 ounces baked tofu, cubed
    4 large eggs (poached, fried, or scrambled)
    ½ cup cashews
    ½ cup sunflower seeds

In a large sauté pan over medium heat, melt the oil. Add the shallot and cook, stirring occasionally, until soft, 3 to 4 minutes. Add the mushrooms, garlic, and salt and sauté until the mushrooms are tender, about 3 minutes. Stir in the peas and continue cooking for another 3 minutes.

Stir in the rice and cook until heated through. Remove from the heat and incorporate the kimchi. Top with your desired protein and enjoy!

BRAIN FOOD FACT

Kimchi is a traditional Korean condiment made by fermenting cabbage and radishes, along with something spicy like chili peppers. It's like sauerkraut with a kick! This is the kind of heat that's good for the gut because it's loaded with probiotics and antioxidants.

Yam and Brussels Sprout Hash with Smoked Salmon

Another name for this dish could be Turn Down the Heat Hash because all of the ingredients that go into the skillet have a way of actively cooling down inflammation. Some featured favorites are the beta-carotene in the yams, the phytonutrients in the brussels sprouts, the volatile oils in the turmeric, and of course the omega-3s in the smoked salmon. The best part is, the flavor combination in this rustic hash can't be beat—sweetness from the yams, buttery goodness from the leeks, and earthy peppery notes from the turmeric all work together to make magic. If you want to amp up the protein and brighten your day, top it with a runny-yolk egg. Perfection!

Makes 6 servings

1 tablespoon extra-virgin olive oil
2 medium leeks, white and light-green
    parts only, rinsed well and sliced
    into half moons
2 cups shredded brussels sprouts
2 cloves garlic, minced
¼ cup water

2 unpeeled garnet yams, cut into
    ¼-inch cubes
2 teaspoons ground turmeric
2 teaspoons ground cumin
1 teaspoon sea salt
1 teaspoon freshly ground black
    pepper
8 ounces smoked salmon, flaked

Preheat the oven to 375 degrees F.

Heat the oil in a large ovenproof skillet with a lid over medium heat. Add the leeks and sauté until they begin to soften, 3 to 4 minutes. Stir in the brussels sprouts, garlic, and water. Cover and let steam for 3 minutes. Stir in the yams, turmeric, cumin, salt, pepper, and salmon.

Transfer the skillet to the oven and roast for 20 to 25 minutes, or until the yams can be easily pierced with a fork.

Quinoa Flapjacks with Cinnamon Cashew Cream

A friend of mine was doing a farm stay and told me about some simple quinoa pancakes that the host would make from grinding quinoa into flour. It struck me as such a simple concept and a great way for someone who's avoiding gluten to be able to enjoy a pancake-style breakfast that's a whole lot more nourishing than some of the gluten-free baking mixes.

Makes 6 servings

FOR THE FLAPJACKS
1 cup quinoa, rinsed and well drained
2 tablespoons chia seeds
1½ teaspoons baking powder
¼ teaspoon baking soda
¼ teaspoon sea salt
1½ cups unsweetened soy or
   almond milk
2 large eggs, lightly beaten
1 pear, peeled and grated

2 tablespoons pure maple syrup
2 teaspoons coconut oil

FOR THE CASHEW CREAM
1 cup raw cashews
2 teaspoons raw honey
2 teaspoons ground cinnamon
½ teaspoon vanilla extract
½ cup water

To make the flapjacks, in a dry skillet over medium heat, toast the quinoa, stirring occasionally, for about 7 minutes. Remove the quinoa from the heat when it starts to make a popping sound. Let it cool for 10 minutes before transferring to a food processor. Add the chia seeds and blend the mixture to a flour consistency.

Transfer the flour to a mixing bowl and whisk in the baking powder, baking soda, and salt. Stir in the soy milk, eggs, pear, and maple syrup, mixing until the ingredients are well blended.

CONTINUED

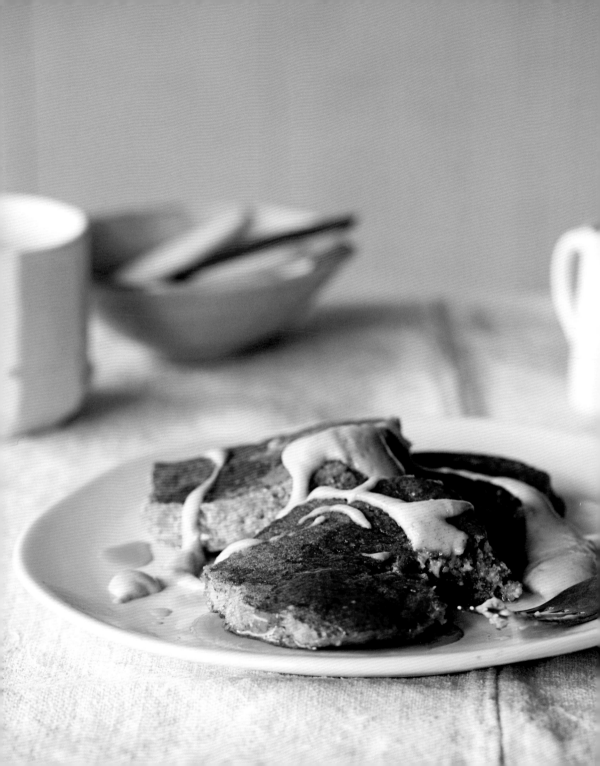

Heat the oil in a large nonstick skillet over medium heat. With a small ladle, scoop about ¼ cup of the flapjack batter into the pan for each flapjack and spread into 3-inch rounds. Cook three flapjacks at a time, being careful not to crowd them. Cook for 1 to 2 minutes, or until bubbles start to form. Flip the flapjacks and cook for another 2 minutes, or until golden brown on both sides. Repeat with the remaining batter.

Meanwhile, make the cashew cream. In a food processor, combine the cashews, honey, cinnamon, and vanilla. With the motor running, slowly add the water and blend until it's the texture of creamy peanut butter.

To serve, place one or two flapjacks on each plate and top with a generous dollop of cashew cream.

For an egg-free version, simply omit the eggs from the batter and allow it to sit for about 10 minutes before cooking.

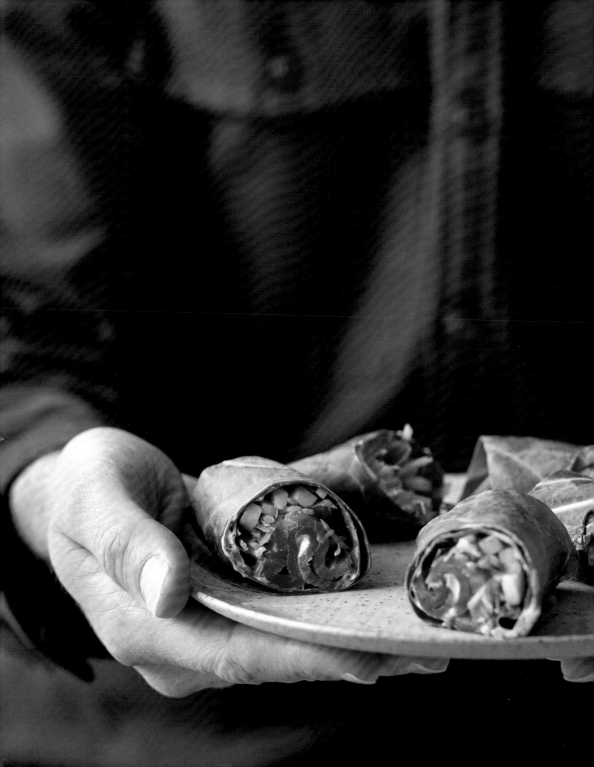

Mood-Boosting Snacks

»»««

We all eat, and it would be a sad waste
of opportunity to eat badly.

—ANNA THOMAS

>> >> << <<

>> >> << <<

Honey-Glazed Walnuts with Cinnamon Spice

DIFFICULTY METER
● ● ● ● ●

Walnuts are hands down the most anti-inflammatory nut among all the tree nuts, and it's probably no accident that they're shaped like a brain since they also appear to be good for cognitive function. Sadly, they rarely make the list of people's favorite nuts to eat. That's likely due to the slight bitterness that comes from the skins, which incidentally contain some of this nut's most powerful antioxidants. Coating walnuts with the sweet-spicy combo of honey, cinnamon, and cayenne makes them absolutely irresistible and universally improves their flavor ranking.

Makes 4 servings

¼ cup raw honey
2 teaspoons ground cinnamon
¼ teaspoon sea salt

⅛ teaspoon ground cayenne
1½ cups walnuts
Coconut oil, for greasing

Preheat the oven to 325 degrees F.

In a small bowl, combine the honey, cinnamon, salt, and cayenne. Mix with a fork until well combined.

In a medium bowl, put the walnuts and drizzle with the honey mixture, carefully stirring with the fork until the walnuts are well coated.

Lightly grease a baking sheet with coconut oil. Spread the walnuts on the baking sheet and bake for 10 minutes, or until they start to turn darker brown. Allow them to cool completely, then break into bite-size pieces. Store in the refrigerator for up to 2 weeks.

BRAIN FOOD FACT

Research shows that walnut consumption in a Mediterranean diet is associated with better memory scores and cognitive function. The results suggest that antioxidants present in walnuts (over other nuts) may help counteract age-related cognitive decline and reduce the incidence of neurodegenerative diseases.

Sassy Punks

Pepitas, shelled pumpkin seeds, are such a fun snack and have a much lighter, crunchier texture than seeds straight out of the pumpkin. Buy them raw in bulk and roast them with any combination of seasonings that appeal to you. I like to spice it up a bit and use some curry powder with turmeric to maximize the anti-inflammatory effect. Be creative—sass it up!

Makes 4 servings

1 cup raw pepitas (shelled
  pumpkin seeds)
2 teaspoons extra-virgin olive oil
1 teaspoon curry powder

¾ teaspoon sea salt
½ teaspoon granulated garlic
½ teaspoon sweet paprika
⅛ teaspoon ground cayenne

Preheat the oven to 325 degrees F.

In a medium bowl, combine all the ingredients and toss until the pepitas are well coated. Spread on a baking sheet and bake, stirring occasionally, for 10 to 12 minutes, or until lightly toasted.

BRAIN FOOD FACT

Pumpkin seeds are a very good source of zinc, which is required for the production of GABA, a neurotransmitter that's key for that calm, cool, and collected feeling.

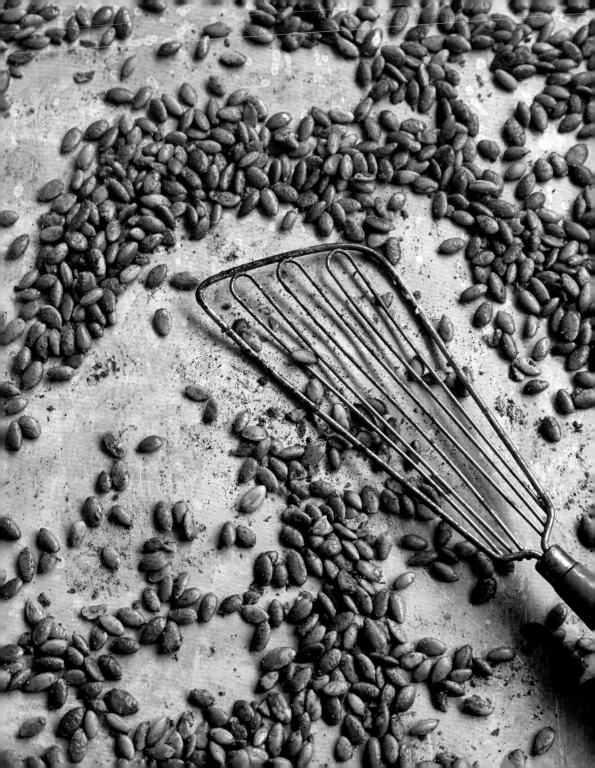

Almond-Coconut Bites

Clients always ask me for healthy, portable snack ideas. These truffle-like snack bites are perfect for the person or family on the go. They also serve as a quick fix when sugar cravings are feeling out of control. The sweetness from the dates and cinnamon, along with the hint of chocolate from the cocoa nibs, will give you the impression you're indulging in a candy bar (but with none of the guilt).

Makes 12 servings

2 cups raw almonds
1 tablespoon ground cinnamon
⅛ teaspoon sea salt
7 Medjool dates, pitted

3 tablespoons cocoa nibs
½ cup unsweetened shredded coconut

In a food processor, process the almonds, cinnamon, and salt until the nuts are finely ground, about 1 minute. Add the dates and process again until well combined; the mixture should have a thick, sticky consistency. Pulse in the cocoa nibs. Check to see if you can form a ball by rolling some of the mixture in your hands. If it falls apart easily, add another date or two.

Spread the coconut on a plate. Scoop the nut mixture with a large spoon and roll into 1-inch balls. Roll the balls in the coconut until they are generously coated. Store the truffles in the refrigerator for up to 1 week or freeze for up to 6 months.

BRAIN FOOD FACT

Of all the nuts, almonds are a superior source of mood-enhancing amino acids like tryptophan, threonine, and tyrosine.

Sunny Oat Squares

Whenever I run a half marathon, my pre-run breakfast is a peanut butter–oat bar I discovered at Great Harvest Bread Company. It always gives me the perfect amount of slow-release energy to get through the run. That's what inspired these tasty delights. I love the flavor of sunflower seed butter, and it makes me happy that these squares are peanut and tree nut free so they're a low allergy snack that's "safe" for kids to take to school or share as a healthy post-game snack with their teammates.

Makes 6 servings

⅔ cup natural sunflower seed butter (I like SunButter Natural)
⅓ cup raw honey or pure maple syrup
½ cup unsweetened shredded coconut

1¼ cups rolled oats
¼ cup unsweetened dried fruit (e.g., raisins, cherries, apple juice–sweetened cranberries)
1 teaspoon coconut oil

In a large bowl, combine the sunflower butter and honey and mix well.

In a small sauté pan over medium-low heat, toast the coconut, stirring frequently, until it begins to turn golden brown, 2 to 3 minutes. Transfer to the bowl with the sunflower butter and honey. Stir in the oats and dried fruit until all ingredients are thoroughly combined.

Lightly grease an 8-inch square baking dish. Transfer the oat mixture to the dish and spread in an even layer. Refrigerate for at least 1 hour, then cut into six squares. Wrap each one individually in plastic wrap for a grab-and-go snack. Store in the refrigerator for up to 2 weeks.

Avocado Boats with Shrimp Aboard

DIFFICULTY METER

Talk about the ultimate easy brain-food snack! This recipe takes mere minutes to assemble and uses ingredients that are acclaimed for stabilizing mood and promoting good rest. The fresh kraut brings some probiotics on board, which makes the gut happy and the brain relaxed. I've recommended this be eaten a couple hours before bed, after a light dinner, with good results. Clients come back and tell me that sleep comes easier and they look forward to indulging in this savory, satisfying snack in the evening. Some even say it helps eliminate mindless late-night grazing.

Makes 4 servings

½ pound peeled cooked baby shrimp
2 heaping tablespoons sauerkraut or
   other favorite fermented vegetable

½ teaspoon sea salt
2 ripe avocados, halved

In a small mixing bowl, combine the shrimp, sauerkraut, and salt and stir well. Scoop the mixture into the avocado halves, piling it on generously, and enjoy!

BRAIN FOOD FACT

Shrimp are an excellent source of tryptophan, that lovely little sleepy-time amino acid. Just 3 ounces provides over 100 percent of the daily value. Shrimp are also rich in minerals, such as iron and zinc, that help ward off depression.

Edamame Guacamole with Crudités

If you're suffering from hummus fatigue, here's a tasty new twist that's bound to get you excited about dipping vegetables again. I realize that guacamole purists might take exception to the notion of adding sweet green soybeans to the mix, but blending in the edamame gives the guacamole a heartier texture and considerably elevates the nutritional profile of this tasty snack. When I serve this as an appetizer at parties, I like to scoop it into little cordial glasses and arrange some matchstick vegetables in each glass.

Makes 6 servings

1 avocado, halved

1 cup frozen shelled edamame, thawed or lightly steamed

3 tablespoons extra-virgin olive oil, plus more if needed

2 tablespoons gluten-free tamari

1 tablespoon freshly squeezed lemon juice

1 tablespoon ground turmeric

2 teaspoons ground cumin

1 teaspoon sea salt

Assorted fresh vegetables (e.g., carrots, snap peas, jicama, cucumbers, peppers, radishes), thinly sliced, for dipping

Scoop the avocado into a food processor or blender. Add the edamame, oil, tamari, lemon juice, turmeric, cumin, and salt and blend until smooth and creamy. Incorporate additional oil for a smoother texture.

Serve with assorted vegetables—the more color, the better!

TIME-SAVING TIP

This can be the perfect afternoon snack to ward off the dreaded 3 p.m. energy dip. Chop up the vegetables in advance (or buy precut) and place them in a gallon freezer bag. Pack up 1½ cups of the dip and take it to work Monday morning with the bag of vegetables. Now you've got your afternoon snack taken care of for the whole workweek!

Truffled Eggs

I'm a fan of deviled eggs but have always considered them to be somewhat boring. I took a cue from Anne Burrell on the Food Network channel and added some truffle oil to my eggs. That was definitely a game changer, but then I also thought it might be fun (and healthier) to use hummus and a little bit of olive oil instead of mayo. This is definitely a jazzed-up version of the classic deviled egg, and it's a hit at every party. Chopped kalamata olives blended into the filling make a nice addition if you're so inclined.

Makes 12 egg halves

6 large eggs
1 cup creamy hummus (store-bought
   is fine)
2 tablespoons extra-virgin olive oil

2 teaspoons truffle oil
1 tablespoon ground turmeric
⅛ teaspoon ground cayenne

Place the eggs in a medium pot and fill it with tap water until the eggs are completely covered. Bring the water to a gentle but steady boil then immediately turn off the heat. Cover and let the eggs sit for exactly 13 minutes. Drain the water and run the eggs under cold water or refrigerate until ready to use.

Peel the eggs and cut in half lengthwise. Scoop the yolks into a medium mixing bowl and mash them with a fork. Add the hummus, oils, turmeric, and cayenne and whisk with the fork until well blended and smooth.

Spoon the yolk mixture into the whites and refrigerate until ready to serve.

TIME SAVING TIP

The shake-and-peel method is my favorite for peeling multiple hard-boiled eggs. After you run the eggs under cold water and drain them, start shaking the pot vigorously, *like you mean it*! Run cold water back into the pot to cover the eggs and then gently squeeze the submerged eggs out of their shells.

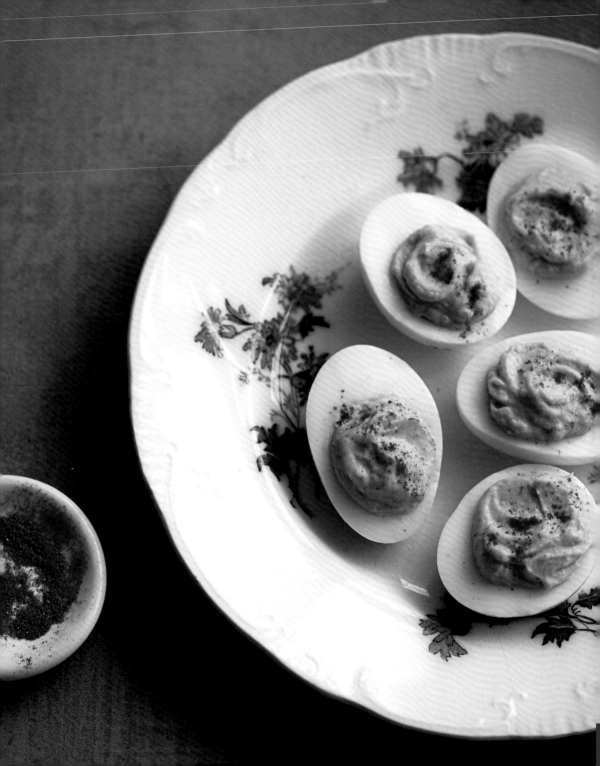

Roasted Roots Bathed in Balsamic

When fall and winter approach, I've noticed there's a natural tendency for people in our cooler Northwest climate to be a little less enthusiastic about munching on raw vegetables throughout the day. Roasting vegetables gives them such a pleasant, sweet flavor and softens the cool crunch of their raw counterparts.

Makes 6 servings

1 medium garnet yam, chopped into 1-inch chunks

2 turnips, chopped into 1-inch chunks

1 large rutabaga, chopped into 1-inch chunks

3 medium crimson beets or Chioggia beets, scrubbed, trimmed, and chopped into 1-inch chunks

2 tablespoons grapeseed or sunflower oil

1 teaspoon coarse sea salt

3 tablespoons balsamic vinegar

2 tablespoons extra-virgin olive oil

3 tablespoons black sesame seeds

1 tablespoon dried Italian herbs

Preheat the oven to 425 degree F.

In a large bowl, toss the yam, turnips, rutabaga, and beets. Drizzle with the grapeseed oil, sprinkle with the salt, and mix until well coated.

Spread the vegetables in a single layer on a large baking sheet or preheated pizza stone. Roast for 20 minutes, stirring halfway through. Transfer the vegetables back to the large bowl.

Drizzle the vinegar and olive oil over the vegetables, and stir in sesame seeds and Italian herbs. Transfer to single-serving containers for easy grab-and-go snacks that can be eaten cold or quickly warmed.

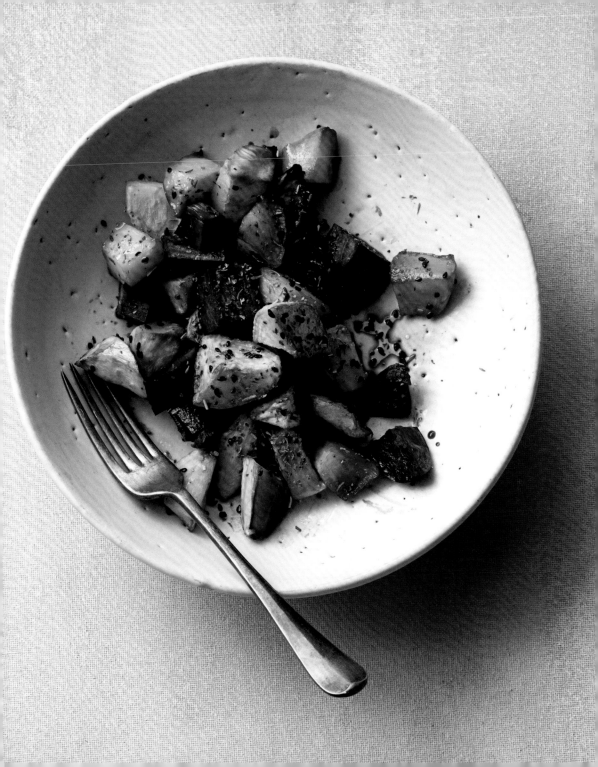

Spicy Tahini Tofu Bites

DIFFICULTY METER
● ● ● ● ● ●

Tofu is such a perfect plant-based source of protein, but sometimes it still gets a bad rap for being kind of "blah." With the combination of tahini, lime juice, ginger, and red pepper flakes, no one will accuse these tofu bites of being boring. I encourage clients to make these on the weekend and take a container to work to balance out an afternoon snack, or to throw on a salad when lunch is lacking in protein.

Makes 6 servings

¼ cup tahini
¼ cup full-fat, unsweetened
    coconut milk
2 tablespoons freshly squeezed
    lime juice
½ teaspoon freshly grated lime zest

1 clove garlic, minced
¾ teaspoon crushed red pepper flakes
½ teaspoon fresh ginger, minced
1 pound extra-firm tofu (I prefer
    Wildwood organic sprouted
    tofu), drained

Preheat the oven to 350 degrees F.

In an 8-inch square baking dish, whisk together the tahini, coconut milk, lime juice and zest, garlic, red pepper flakes, and ginger.

Carefully pat the tofu dry with a paper towel. Cut it into 1-inch cubes, add to the baking dish, and gently stir until the tofu is evenly coated.

Bake the tofu for 1 hour, stirring every 15 minutes. It should be golden brown. Serve warm, or allow it to cool for 15 to 20 minutes before refrigerating for a portable high-protein snack.

BRAIN FOOD FACT

Soy is a good source of folate, magnesium, and iron and an excellent source of tryptophan. It also contains many of the mood-enhancing nutrients that are sometimes more difficult to find in plant-based foods.

Smoked Salmon Roll Ups

Smoky, salty, tangy, creamy, crunchy—oh my! These salmon roll ups awaken the senses and provide the ultimate mindful eating experience. Rarely can you get so much variety in one bite, which is part of what makes these savory snacks so satisfying. It's also the perfect balance of protein, healthy fats, and some complex carbs from the vegetables. Your taste buds will rejoice and your brain will thank you.

Makes 6 servings

¼ cup plain full-fat yogurt
1 tablespoon stone-ground mustard
1 teaspoon raw honey
1 bunch collard greens, stemmed and halved lengthwise

1 (4-ounce) package smoked salmon (lox-style works best)
1 English cucumber, cut into thin matchsticks
1 small red onion, thinly sliced
½ cup shredded carrots

In a small bowl, combine the yogurt, mustard, and honey.

Lay out a collard leaf strip and place a slice of the smoked salmon in the center, then top with a dollop of the dressing. Arrange some cucumber, onion, and carrots in the center and roll the leaf up burrito-style. Repeat until you run out of ingredients. Serve chilled.

BRAIN FOOD FACT

The omega-3s in salmon and the vitamin K in collard greens actively shut down inflammatory signaling, making this the ultimate anti-inflammatory snack.

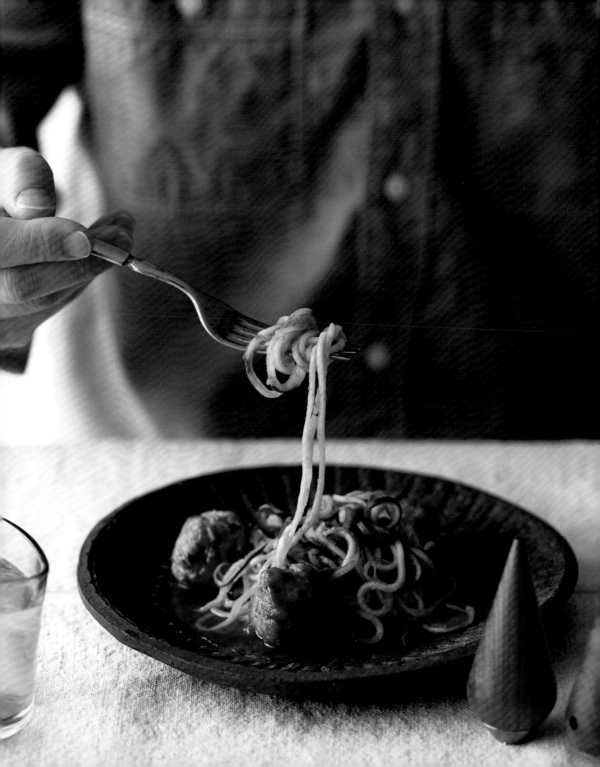

Mind-Altering Main Dishes

»»««

You don't have to cook fancy or complicated masterpieces—just good food from fresh ingredients.

—JULIA CHILD

>> >> << <<

>> >> << <<

Seafood Parchment Packets

Cooking fish in parchment—or as the French say *en papillote*—is one of the easiest cooking methods, and it significantly reduces your chances of drying out the fish. The parchment, when folded correctly, prevents the steam from escaping and seals in the flavor of the fish. When you throw some vegetables in, it can be the equivalent of a one-pot meal. You can carefully fold the parchment back and serve it right in the paper for a rustic look, or slide the fish off the skin, top it with the vegetables, and compost the parchment—no hassle, no mess! The following are some recipes to get you started. Once you get the technique down, you can experiment with endless combinations of ingredients.

Makes 4 servings (each option)

Cut four 10-by-12-inch pieces of parchment paper. Center one fillet, skin side down, on each piece. Arrange the vegetables on either side of the fish. Drizzle the sauce over the fish and vegetables.

Bring two edges of the parchment paper together over the center of the fish and carefully fold them together, rolling down toward the fish but leaving about ½ inch between it and the paper. Then tightly twist the two open ends of the parchment— the packet will look a bit like a candy wrapper. The fillet should be well sealed inside the parchment so no steam escapes. Repeat with the other three packets.

Place the parchment packets on a baking sheet and bake for 15 to 20 minutes, depending on the thickness of the fish.

Carefully open the parchment packets (beware of escaping steam). The cooked fish should be flakey and easily slip off the skin. Transfer it to a plate to serve.

CONTINUED

Whitefish and Broccoli with Lemony Tahini Sauce

¼ cup tahini
¼ cup mushroom or vegetable broth
2 tablespoons freshly squeezed
  lemon juice
1 tablespoon gluten-free tamari
1 clove garlic, minced

½ teaspoon sea salt
1½ pounds whitefish (such as halibut
  or black cod), deboned and cut into
  4 fillets
1 head broccoli, chopped into florets

Preheat the oven to 350 degrees F.

To make the sauce, in a small bowl, whisk together the tahini, broth, lemon juice, tamari, garlic, and salt until smooth and creamy. To cook the fish, follow the parchment packet instructions on page 77.

Rockfish, Mushrooms, and Fennel

1 teaspoon ground cumin
½ teaspoon ground coriander
½ teaspoon sea salt
½ teaspoon ground white pepper

1½ pounds rockfish, deboned and cut
  into 4 fillets
8 shiitake mushrooms, thinly sliced
1 fennel bulb, trimmed and shaved
  into thin slices

Preheat the oven to 350 degrees F.

In a small bowl, combine the cumin, coriander, salt, and pepper. To cook the fish, follow the parchment packet instructions on page 77.

Salmon and Kale with Creamy Coconut Sauce

1 cup full-fat, unsweetened coconut
   milk (I like Aroy-D or Thai Kitchen)
1 tablespoon freshly squeezed
   lemon juice
2 teaspoons dried dill
2 teaspoons dried oregano
1 teaspoon granulated garlic,
   or 2 cloves garlic, minced

½ teaspoon sea salt
1½ pounds salmon, deboned and cut
   into 4 fillets
1 bunch curly kale (such as red
   Russian), stemmed and
   coarsely chopped

Preheat the oven to 350 degrees F.

To make the sauce, in a small bowl, whisk together the coconut milk, lemon juice, dill, oregano, garlic, and salt. To cook the fish, follow the parchment packet instructions on page 77.

BRAIN FOOD FACT

Salmon is a superior source of omega-3 fatty acids, which increase dopamine binding and down-regulate inflammation. Salmon is also an excellent source of tryptophan, making it a great meal for a more restful sleep.

Poached Halibut with Pistachio Pesto

Poaching fish is a foolproof method that eliminates any worry of overcooking and drying out the fish. The fish simply steams in some cooking liquid, and it's easy to tell when it's cooked to perfection because it will flake easily with a fork. I like this recipe best with halibut, but black cod or lingcod work equally well here. This variation on classic pesto has a rich, sweet flavor that comes from using pistachios in place of pine nuts.

Makes 4 servings

2 cups packed fresh basil
¼ cup shelled raw or roasted
   unsalted pistachios
¼ cup extra-virgin olive oil, plus more
   if needed
1¼ cups water, divided
2 cloves garlic

1½ teaspoons sea salt, divided
1 cup vegetable broth
1½ pounds halibut or other whitefish,
   deboned and cut into 4 fillets
½ teaspoon freshly ground black
   pepper

In a food processor or blender, combine the basil, pistachios, oil, ¼ cup of the water, garlic, and ½ teaspoon of the salt and blend until smooth. Drizzle in additional oil for an even smoother texture, if desired. Set aside.

In a cast-iron skillet or deep sauté pan over medium-high heat, bring the broth and remaining 1 cup water to a gentle boil. Place the halibut in the skillet and season with the remaining 1 teaspoon salt and the pepper. Cover and reduce the heat to medium. Poach for 8 to 9 minutes, depending on the thickness of the fish. The halibut should be opaque in the center but still moist.

Carefully transfer the fillets to plates, leaving the skin behind. Top with a generous dollop of the pesto and serve.

TIP: Use any leftover pesto on zucchini noodles or spaghetti squash. It will keep in the refrigerator for up to a week.

Whitefish Tikka Masala

I've always loved tikka masala but have often been put off by some seemingly labor-intensive recipes. I've made a few modifications to the more traditional preparation, the most obvious being replacing chicken with fish. I've also taken the liberty to consolidate some of the complex seasoning. Garam masala and berbere are blends of many spices that are typically used in tikka masala, and the end result is a very complex, rich, tangy sauce that tastes like it has stewed for hours. The lime leaves brighten it up considerably, but if you can't find lime leaves, you can achieve a similar effect by adding the zest from one lime instead.

Makes 4 servings

- 1 (28-ounce) can diced tomatoes
- 4 cloves garlic, minced
- 2 lime leaves
- ½ teaspoon minced fresh ginger
- 1½ teaspoons sea salt
- 1 teaspoon ground turmeric
- 1 teaspoon garam masala

- 1 teaspoon berbere
- 1 pound whitefish (such as cod), skinned and deboned
- ½ cup plain low-fat Greek yogurt (or use ¼ cup full-fat, unsweetened coconut milk for a dairy-free option)
- 2 cups cooked brown rice or quinoa

In a large skillet or Dutch oven set over medium-low heat, stir together the tomatoes, garlic, lime leaves, ginger, salt, turmeric, garam masala, and berbere. Simmer for 10 minutes, stirring occasionally.

Meanwhile, cut the fish into 1-inch cubes. Stir the fish into the sauce, cover, and cook for 8 to 10 minutes, or until the fish is opaque throughout. Discard the lime leaves, stir in the yogurt, and serve over the rice or quinoa.

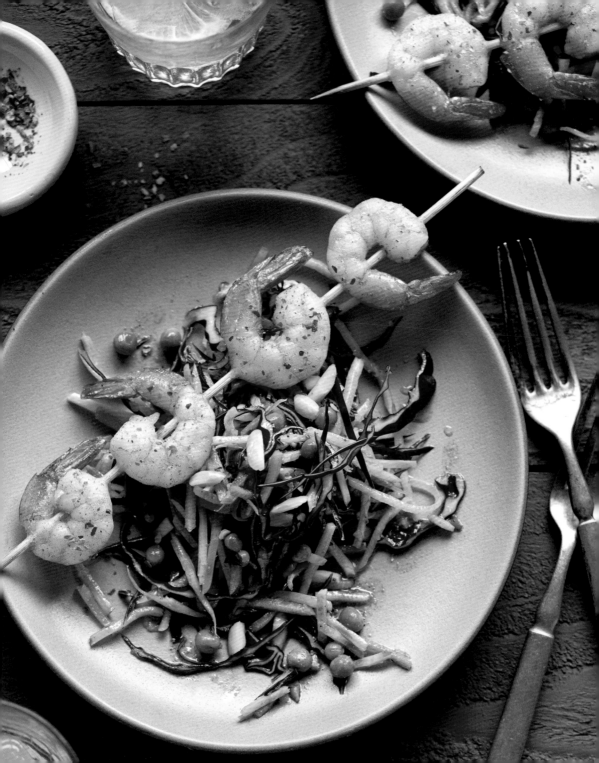

Curried Shrimp Kebabs
with Spring Slaw

Whenever I make curried shrimp, I have the desire to pair it with coleslaw. I enjoy the texture combination—I love how the broccoli and cabbage add some crunch. Broccoli slaw is always fun, but if you can't find it or prefer traditional slaw, using only cabbage is just fine. I've gotten into the habit of shredding the unused stems of my broccoli so I often have a stash on hand to toss with cabbage or sauté with other vegetables.

Makes 4 servings

FOR THE KEBABS
½ cup extra-virgin olive oil
1 clove garlic, minced
1 tablespoon curry powder
½ teaspoon crushed red pepper flakes
½ teaspoon sea salt
1 pound large tail-on shrimp, shelled
   and deveined

FOR THE SLAW
1 (10-ounce) bag broccoli slaw, or
   1 small head green cabbage,
   shredded
½ small head purple cabbage,
   shredded

1 small jicama, peeled and shredded
¾ cup shelled spring peas or frozen
   petite peas, thawed
½ cup slivered almonds
¼ cup walnut oil
3 tablespoons freshly squeezed
   lime juice
1 tablespoon raw honey
   or agave nectar
1 teaspoon ground cumin
½ teaspoon garam masala
¼ teaspoon sea salt

4 or 5 (10-inch) skewers, soaked in
   water for 20 minutes

Preheat the oven to 400 degrees F.

In a medium bowl, whisk together the olive oil, garlic, curry powder, red pepper flakes, and salt. Add the shrimp and toss until well coated. Marinate for 20 to 30 minutes.

CONTINUED

Meanwhile, make the slaw. In a large bowl, combine the broccoli, cabbage, jicama, peas, and almonds. In a small bowl, whisk together the walnut oil, lime juice, honey, cumin, garam masala, and salt. Drizzle the dressing over the slaw and toss until well coated.

Thread the shrimp onto the presoaked skewers and arrange the skewers on a baking sheet. Bake for 8 to 10 minutes, or until the shrimp are opaque throughout.

Place a generous scoop of slaw in the center of each plate and lay a shrimp skewer across the top. Garnish with lime wedges, if desired.

BRAIN FOOD FACT

Shrimp are an excellent source of tryptophan, with just three ounces providing over 100 percent of the daily value. They're also rich in minerals that are essential for warding off depression, such as iron and zinc.

Seafood and White Bean Cassoulet

A traditional French cassoulet is a rich, slow-cooked casserole that's loaded with meat (typically pork and often duck). This updated take on the French classic is still rich and delicious, but the meat is replaced with more anti-inflammatory, brain-boosting seafood. This is my favorite Sunday supper and also a big hit at dinner parties. The white beans and unique blend of spices give it a wonderfully complex flavor that has a gourmet feel without requiring you to spend hours in the kitchen.

Makes 6 servings

1 tablespoon extra-virgin olive oil
1 small yellow onion, chopped
1 carrot, chopped
1 stalk celery, chopped
1 cup shredded savoy cabbage
2 cloves garlic, minced
1 (28-ounce) can diced tomatoes
1 (15-ounce) can cannellini beans, rinsed and drained
1½ cups fish stock
½ pound medium shrimp, peeled and deveined

½ pound bay scallops
½ pound wild-caught salmon, skinned, deboned, and cut into 1-inch chunks
2 tablespoons tomato paste
1 tablespoon minced fresh oregano, or 1 teaspoon dried
1 tablespoon fresh thyme leaves, or 1 teaspoon dried
1½ teaspoons sea salt
1 teaspoon ground white pepper
1 bay leaf
Juice from ½ lemon

Preheat the oven to 350 degrees F.

In a Dutch oven over medium heat, add the oil and onion. Sauté for 5 minutes, or until the onion is translucent. Stir in the carrot and celery and cook for another 5 minutes. Add the cabbage, garlic, tomatoes, beans, stock, shrimp, scallops, salmon, tomato paste, oregano, thyme, salt, pepper, and bay leaf to the pot, cover with a tight-fitting lid, and transfer to the oven. Bake for 25 to 30 minutes, or until the seafood is cooked through. Squeeze the lemon juice over the top, ladle into bowls, and serve.

Slow-Cooked Chicken and White Bean Stew with Rainbow Quinoa

This is one of those one-pot meals that's a universal hit. It's also a good example of how you can use a small amount of poultry surrounded with anti-inflammatory vegetables and herbs to make it pleasing for those who don't feel like a meal is complete without some animal protein.

Makes 6 servings

- 2 large boneless, skinless chicken breasts
- 2 parsnips, chopped
- 2 carrots, chopped
- 1 small white onion, chopped
- 1 stalk celery, chopped
- 1 cup chopped cremini mushrooms
- 5 cloves garlic
- ½ cup rainbow quinoa, rinsed and drained
- 3 tablespoons dried Italian herbs
- 2 teaspoons sea salt
- 1 teaspoon freshly ground black pepper
- 4 cups chicken broth
- 1 (15-ounce) can cannellini beans
- 1 bunch Swiss chard, stemmed and chopped

In a slow cooker, place the chicken, parsnips, carrots, onion, celery, mushrooms, garlic, quinoa, Italian herbs, salt, and pepper. Add the broth and enough water to completely cover the chicken breasts and vegetables (typically about 2 cups). Cover and cook on low for 6 to 7 hours.

Use two forks to shred the chicken breasts right in the slow cooker. Stir until the shredded chicken is well distributed and add the cannellini beans.

Place a handful of chard in the bottom of six bowls, ladle the stew on top, and serve.

TIME-SAVING TIP

Chop the parsnips, carrots, onion, celery, and mushrooms the evening before so you can just dump the ingredients into your slow cooker right before you head off to work.

Sweet-and-Spicy Chicken Chili

If you're looking for the perfect game-day dish, this chili really fits the bill. It's thick and hearty (and healthy, but shhh, they'll never notice). The sweetness from the yams helps balance the heat from the ancho chili and chili powder. This is a great one to make the day before a tailgating party because it gives the flavors time to meld and will deliver even more of a punch after marinating overnight.

Makes 8 servings

1 tablespoon coconut oil
1 small red onion, diced
1 pound ground chicken
2 cloves garlic, minced
3 cups vegetable broth
1 (28-ounce) can diced fire-roasted
  tomatoes
1 (15-ounce) can black beans
1 (15-ounce) can adzuki beans
1 medium garnet yam, peeled and cut
  into ½-inch cubes

1 ancho chili, seeded and diced
1 tablespoon ground cumin
2 teaspoons chili powder
2 teaspoons ground turmeric
1 teaspoon sea salt
½ teaspoon ground cinnamon
1 bunch Tuscan kale, stemmed and
  finely chopped
1 avocado, sliced

Heat the oil in a stockpot or Dutch oven over medium heat. Add the onion and cook for about 5 minutes, or until translucent. Add the chicken and garlic, breaking up the meat with a spatula. Sauté until the chicken is cooked through, about 8 minutes. Add the broth, tomatoes, beans, yam, and chili pepper. Stir in the cumin, chili powder, turmeric, salt, and cinnamon and simmer for 20 to 25 minutes, or until the yams are soft. Fold in the kale and cook for another 10 minutes.

Ladle the chili into bowls, top with avocado slices, and serve.

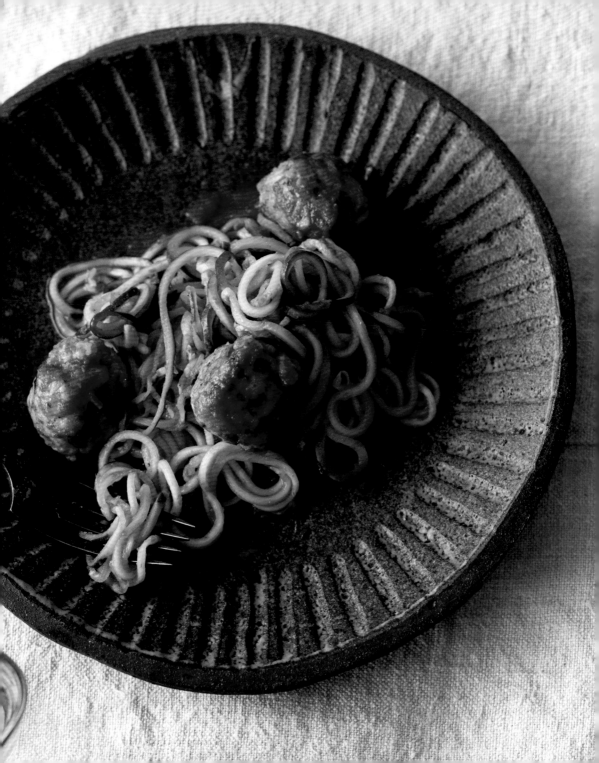

Zoodles Marinara with Turkey Meatballs

I'm always on a quest to develop family-friendly recipes that kids enjoy and parents can feel good about eating. This is obviously a healthier take on spaghetti and meatballs, but it's also a way to get at least six different vegetables into a meal without anyone objecting. I often add finely chopped kale to the meatballs, which goes undetected. Feel free to be creative and use the meatballs as a delivery system for a variety of shredded vegetables. You can also blend vegetables into the marinara sauce if you have the kind of picky eaters who can detect a speck of green in their food from a mile away.

Makes 4 servings

1 tablespoon extra-virgin olive oil
1 small yellow onion, diced
6 cremini mushrooms, finely chopped
1½ teaspoon sea salt, divided
1 clove garlic, minced
1 pound ground turkey
1 egg, lightly beaten
1 carrot, shredded
¼ cup rolled oats

2 tablespoons dried parsley
2 teaspoons dried tarragon
1 teaspoon dried sage
3 medium zucchini
1 tablespoon grapeseed or
    sunflower oil
1 (18-ounce) jar marinara sauce (no
    sugar added)

Preheat the oven to 375 degrees F.

Heat the olive oil in a cast-iron skillet or Dutch oven over medium heat and add the onion. Sauté for about 5 minutes, or until the onion starts to soften. Add the mushrooms and ½ teaspoon of the salt and sauté for another 3 minutes. Stir in the garlic and remove from the heat.

CONTINUED

In a large bowl, combine the turkey, egg, carrot, and oats. Add the sautéed mushroom mixture, the remaining 1 teaspoon salt, the parsley, tarragon, and sage. Use your hands to knead the ingredients together until well combined. Roll the mixture into small (1-inch) meatballs.

Cut the ends off the zucchini and use a peeler to shave them into noodle-like strips (or use a spiral vegetable slicer).

Wipe out the skillet and return to medium-high heat. Heat the grapeseed oil for 1 minute, until very hot. Carefully arrange the meatballs in the skillet and cook for 2 minutes. Turn and cook for another 2 minutes, and continue turning until the meatballs appear to be evenly cooked on the outside. Add the zucchini noodles (zoodles) to the pan and pour the marinara over the top.

Transfer the skillet to the oven and bake for 20 minutes, or until the meatballs are cooked through.

TIME-SAVING TIP

If you don't want to deal with making the meatballs, you can do a fast and easy deconstructed version of this recipe. Skip the egg and oats and simply sauté the rest of the contents of the meatballs together in a skillet. Add the zoodles and sauce and bake as directed.

Lamb-Stuffed Red Peppers

The thought of stuffed peppers takes me straight back to Grandma's house, where it was commonplace to have green peppers stuffed with hamburger and tomato sauce. While that still brings back fond memories, these are *not* your grandmother's stuffed peppers. We're using the sweeter, antioxidant-rich red bell peppers, and the filling is a savory combo of ground lamb, butternut squash, peas, and parsley. Oh, and it also serves as a great way to hide some chopped kale. You'll never even know it's in there! Be sure to make some extra for leftovers. They're easy to heat and eat for lunch and they also freeze well.

Makes 4 servings

1 pound ground lamb
2 shallots, diced
2 cloves garlic, minced
1 tablespoon dried oregano, or
    3 tablespoons fresh oregano
½ teaspoon sea salt
½ teaspoon freshly ground black
    pepper

1½ cups frozen cubed butternut
    squash
1 cup stemmed and finely chopped
    Tuscan kale
¾ cup frozen petite peas
¼ cup chopped Italian parsley
4 medium red bell peppers

Preheat the oven to 425 degrees F.

In a large ovenproof skillet (cast-iron works great) over medium-high heat, sauté the lamb, breaking it up with a spatula. When the lamb starts to brown, add the shallots, garlic, oregano, salt, and pepper and sauté for 1 to 2 minutes. Add squash, kale, peas, and parsley and sauté for another 2 minutes. Remove the skillet from the heat.

Cut the tops off the bell peppers and scrape out the seeds. Scoop the lamb mixture into the cavities, filling each pepper to the top. Place the peppers into the skillet and transfer to the oven. Bake for 30 minutes, or until the pepper flesh can be easily pierced with a fork.

Slow-Cooked Beef, Broccoli, and Mushroom Stew

There's no vegetable better suited for hanging out with beef than broccoli. This is a hearty stew with layers of flavor; all of the herbs and spices in this dish have potent anti-inflammatory properties, but the best part is how well they complement the beef and broccoli. The mushrooms lend that earthy, umami quality that makes it hard to put down your spoon.

Makes 6 to 8 servings

¼ cup rice flour

3 teaspoons sea salt

¼ teaspoon freshly ground black pepper

3 tablespoons sunflower or grapeseed oil, divided

1 pound grass-fed beef chuck, trimmed of fat and cut into ½-inch cubes

3 cups beef bone broth or mushroom broth

2 tablespoons tomato paste

2 parsnips, chopped

1 yellow onion, diced

1 cup chopped cremini mushrooms

1 teaspoon ground black mustard seeds

1 teaspoon granulated garlic

1 teaspoon ground cumin

1 teaspoon ground turmeric

1 teaspoon ground fennel seed

1 teaspoon chili powder

½ teaspoon ground coriander

¼ teaspoon ground cinnamon

¼ teaspoon ground ginger

1 head broccoli, separated into florets

In a shallow dish, whisk together the flour, salt, and pepper. Heat 2 tablespoons of the oil in a medium skillet over medium-high heat. Dredge the beef cubes in the flour mixture and place them in the skillet. Cook for 5 to 7 minutes, turning occasionally, until the beef begins to brown.

In a slow cooker, gently whisk together the broth, tomato paste, and any remaining flour mixture. Add the browned beef, parsnips, onion, mushrooms, and all of the spices. Cook on low for 8 hours.

Add the broccoli, cook on low for another 30 minutes, and serve.

STORAGE TIP

This stew freezes well and can be kept for 4 to 6 months. Allow the stew to cool for about 1 hour, transfer to glass containers (I use mason jars) leaving ½ inch of headspace, label, and stock the freezer. You'll be delighted to pull out a jar when you come home after a long day and you're not in the mood to cook!

Mock Moussaka

Mashed potatoes replace the traditional béchamel sauce here, but this dish is still rich enough to hold its own. There's something about this combination of textures and the layering of ingredients that reminds me of comforting casseroles from my childhood, but it's definitely a more sophisticated version than any meat-and-potato casserole I ever ate. Fresh ground lamb has such a nice flavor profile and really elevates the richness of this dish.

Makes 8 servings

4 large white potatoes, peeled and
 cut into 2-inch chunks
4 cloves garlic, smashed
1 cup vegetable broth
3 teaspoons sea salt, divided
½ teaspoon freshly ground black
 pepper
1 pound ground lamb
1 teaspoon minced fresh ginger
½ teaspoon ground cinnamon
¼ teaspoon ground allspice
⅛ teaspoon ground cayenne

1 yellow onion, diced
4 cloves garlic, minced
1 cup stemmed and finely chopped
 curly kale (such as red Russian)
¼ cup chopped Italian parsley
1 (28-ounce) can diced tomatoes
2 tablespoons tomato paste
1 tablespoon extra-virgin olive oil
2 small eggplants, cut into
 ¼-inch slices
1 zucchini, cut into ¼-inch slices

In a stockpot, place the potatoes and smashed garlic and cover with water. Bring to a boil over high heat. Reduce the heat to medium and cook for 10 minutes, or until the potatoes are soft. Strain and reserve the cooking liquid. Using electric beaters, mash the potatoes and garlic in the pot, gradually adding the broth, 1 teaspoon of the salt, and pepper. Add reserved cooking liquid as needed to achieve the desired texture. The mixture should be thick enough to hold its form.

Preheat the oven to 350 degrees F.

In a large skillet with a lid over medium heat, sauté the lamb, breaking it up with a spatula. Add 1 teaspoon of the salt, the ginger, cinnamon, allspice, and cayenne and cook for 5 minutes. Add the onion and minced garlic and cook for another 5 minutes, or until the onion softens. Stir in the kale, parsley, tomatoes, tomato paste, and the remaining 1 teaspoon salt. Cover and simmer for 10 minutes.

Drizzle the oil in a 9-by-13-inch baking dish to coat the bottom. Arrange a layer of eggplant and top with half of the lamb mixture. Spread a thin layer of the mashed potatoes and top with a layer of zucchini. Add another layer of the lamb mixture and a second layer of eggplant. Spread the remaining potatoes over the top, making sure to cover the filling completely. Bake for 50 to 60 minutes, or until the top is browned.

Tofu Taco Salad

The trick to getting around any texture objections to tofu is to crumble it and sauté it with a savory seasoning until it starts to get slightly crispy. Tossing it into some greens with crunchy cabbage and dressing it up with salsa and avocado makes it even more irresistible. When I make this taco salad, I like to cook up some extra tofu with the taco seasoning to throw into a bowl of brown rice and vegetables for lunch the next day.

Makes 4 servings

1 tablespoon grapeseed or sunflower oil

1 (15-ounce) package extra-firm tofu

2 tablespoons taco seasoning (I prefer Frontier's all-natural blend)

4 cups mixed greens

1 cup shredded purple cabbage

1 red onion, diced

1 avocado, cut into 1-inch chunks

¾ cup salsa

2 tablespoons extra-virgin olive oil

1 lime, quartered

Heat the oil in a sauté pan over medium-high heat. Wrap the tofu in a large paper towel and gently squeeze to remove excess water. Crumble the tofu and add it to the pan. Sprinkle with the taco seasoning and stir until the tofu is well coated. Sauté for 3 to 4 minutes, stirring frequently, until the tofu starts to get crisp edges.

In a large bowl, toss the greens, cabbage, onion, avocado, salsa, and olive oil. Divide the salad among four plates, top with the tofu, and squeeze fresh lime juice over each salad.

BRAIN FOOD FACT

Soy is a good source of vitamin K and omega-3s, which reduce inflammation. It's an excellent source of tryptophan and contains many of the mood-enhancing nutrients that are sometimes more difficult to find in plant-based foods.

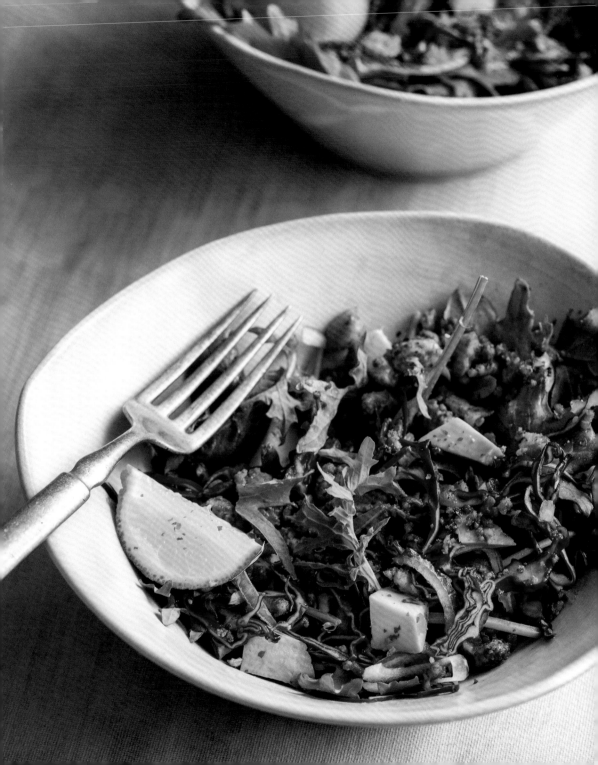

Spaghetti Squash Carbonara with Sautéed Vegetables

The first time I experimented with this recipe I had my doubts. Carbonara is known for being an extremely rich sauce, and while it's mostly eggs, there's generally some form of cream or cheese and a salty meat like ham involved. I wondered if omitting the dairy and the meat and using squash instead of pasta would just be too much of a departure from the original. I needn't have worried: the feedback I got was overwhelmingly positive. The combination of flavors from the mushroom, sun-dried tomatoes, and herbs makes most people forget about what's "missing."

Makes 4 servings

1 cup water
1 medium spaghetti squash, halved lengthwise
1 tablespoon extra-virgin olive oil
1 small white onion, diced
6 cremini mushrooms, chopped
2 cloves garlic, minced
½ teaspoon freshly ground black pepper
1 teaspoon sea salt, divided

¼ cup oil-packed sun-dried tomatoes, drained and chopped
2 cups stemmed and chopped Tuscan kale
2 large eggs
1 tablespoon dried Italian herbs
1 tablespoon nutritional yeast or grated Parmesan
½ teaspoon sea salt

Preheat the oven to 375 degrees F.

Pour the water into a 9-by-13-inch baking dish. Place the squash cut sides down in the dish. Cover tightly with foil and bake for 45 to 50 minutes, or until the squash is tender.

Meanwhile, in a large skillet over medium heat, add the oil and onion. Sauté for 5 minutes, or until the onion is translucent. Stir in the mushrooms, garlic, pepper, and ½ teaspoons of the salt and cook for another 5 minutes. Stir in the sun-dried tomatoes, fold in the kale, and sauté the vegetables for 3 to 5 minutes, or until the kale is slightly wilted. Remove from the heat.

In a small bowl, add the eggs, Italian herbs, nutritional yeast, and the remaining ½ teaspoon salt and whisk until frothy.

Return the skillet to medium heat. While the squash is still warm, scoop out and discard the seeds, then shred the flesh with a fork. Scoop the flesh into the skillet and stir to incorporate. Turn off the heat and pour in the egg mixture, stirring briskly until the eggs thicken (do not let them scramble). Serve immediately.

BRAIN FOOD FACT

Eggs are one of the best food sources of choline, which helps boost memory and improves cognitive function. As an added bonus, high-choline foods may help decrease anxiety, some studies show.

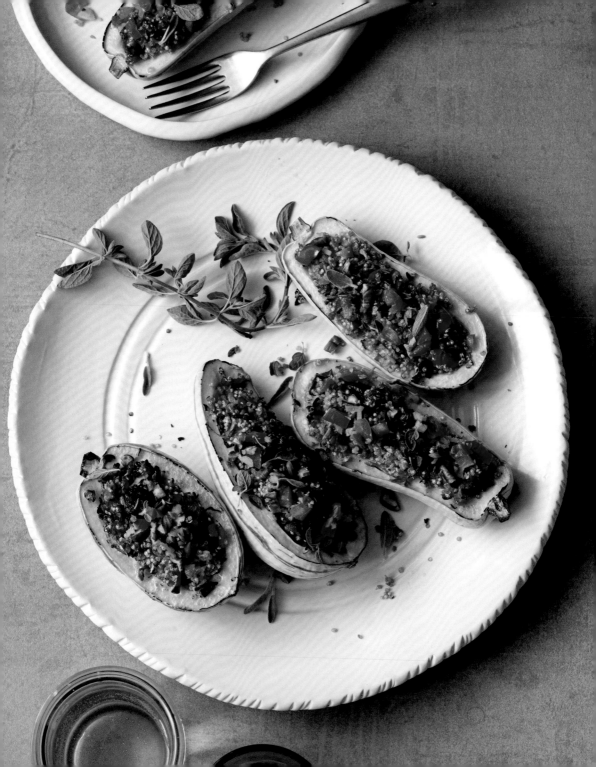

Delicata Squash with Quinoa-Pecan Stuffing

I love vegetarian dishes that feel hearty enough to make you forget that you're not eating meat. This is one of those dishes. The quinoa stuffing, dressed up with pecans and seasoned with sage, is reminiscent of a Thanksgiving meal. The delicata squash is the perfect reservoir for the quinoa filling. It lends a sweet, rich flavor and a meaty texture, plus the skin is tender enough to make the entire container edible.

Makes 6 servings

2 cups vegetable broth
1 cup quinoa, rinsed and drained
1 tablespoon extra-virgin olive oil
1 small onion, diced
¾ cup chopped cremini mushrooms
1 carrot, shredded
1 red bell pepper, chopped

1 clove garlic, minced
1 teaspoon dried sage
1 teaspoon dried oregano
½ cup finely chopped pecans
2 teaspoons sea salt
3 medium delicata squashes,
    halved lengthwise

In a medium saucepan over medium-high heat, combine the broth and quinoa and bring to a boil. Reduce the heat to low, cover, and simmer for 20 minutes without stirring. Fluff with a fork and let cool for about 5 minutes.

Preheat the oven to 350 degrees F.

In a large sauté pan over medium heat, add the oil and onion and sauté until translucent, about 5 minutes. Stir in the mushrooms and sauté for 2 minutes. Add the carrot, bell pepper, garlic, sage, and oregano and sauté for another 3 minutes. Stir in the quinoa, pecans, and salt.

Scoop the seeds and stringy pulp out of the squash halves. Arrange the squashes cut side up in shallow baking dish and generously fill them with the quinoa stuffing. Cover the dish with foil and bake for 25 to 30 minutes, or until the squashes are tender.

Slow-Cooked Lentil and Quinoa Stew

Whenever I think of hearty vegetarian stews, my mind immediately goes to lentils. There's something about them that just has a "meaty" quality. The French lentils are my favorite because they don't disintegrate when cooked. Some of the other brown and green lentils would work just fine too. Adding quinoa to the stew guarantees a satiating dish that's more nutritionally complete. The seasoning blend has an Indian flair and can be fiddled with if you like more heat.

Makes 8 servings

2½ cups water
2½ cups vegetable or
    mushroom broth
¾ cup French green lentils
½ cup quinoa, rinsed and drained
2 cups diced tomatoes (canned is OK)
1 cup chopped cremini mushrooms
1 small white onion, chopped

3 carrots, diced
2 stalks celery, diced
4 cloves garlic, minced
2 tablespoons ground turmeric
2 tablespoons ground cumin
1 tablespoon sea salt
2 teaspoons sweet paprika
1 teaspoon crushed red pepper flakes

In a slow cooker, combine all the ingredients and stir well. Cover and cook on low for 6 to 7 hours.

TIME-SAVING TIP

Chop the mushrooms, onion, carrots, celery, and garlic the evening before, so you can just dump the ingredients into your slow cooker right before you head off to work. If you're really pressed for time, some stores sell mirepoix, which is a prechopped combo of onion, carrot, and celery (you'll need about 1½ cups), and you can also purchase presliced mushrooms.

Beans, Greens, and Grains Bowls

DIFFICULTY METER
● ● ● ● ● ●

This magical trio of ingredients is my versatile go-to for a nutritionally balanced, supersatisfying vegetarian meal. The best part is, there's a virtually endless number of combinations you can use, so you'll never get bored with one bowl. Here are some ingredients to mix and match:

BEANS	GREENS	GRAINS	ADDITIONS
Black beans	Spinach	Quinoa	Salsa
Chickpeas	Chard	Brown rice	Guacamole
Adzuki beans	Kale	Bhutanese red rice	Pesto
Shelled edamame	Collards	Wild rice	Olive oil and basil
Cannellini beans	Broccoli	Millet	Garlic sauce
Black-eyed peas	Bok choy		Toasted sesame oil
Lentils			Chopped fresh herbs

The five recipes that follow are a few of my favorite ways to combine beans, greens, and grains, but don't let that stop you from experimenting with countless other variations!

Makes 4 servings (each option)

CONTINUED

Southwestern Burrito Bowl

2 cups vegetable broth
1 cup quinoa, rinsed and drained
2 cups spinach or baby kale, chopped
1 (15-ounce) can black beans, rinsed
  and drained
½ cup chopped fire-roasted
  peppers packed in oil, with
  ¼ cup oil reserved

½ cup frozen corn niblets, thawed
1 (4-ounce) can diced green chilies
¼ cup salsa or pico de gallo
¼ cup pepitas (shelled
  pumpkin seeds)
1 avocado, sliced

In a medium saucepan over high heat, combine the broth and quinoa and bring to a boil. Cover, reduce the heat to low, and simmer for 15 to 20 minutes without stirring. Measure 1 cup of the quinoa for use in the salad and save the rest for an easy leftover side dish.

In a large bowl, combine the quinoa, spinach, beans, peppers, corn, and chilies. Drizzle with the oil from the peppers and add the salsa. Toss until well combined. Top with the pepitas and avocado and serve.

Mediterranean Pesto Bowl

2 cups vegetable broth
1 cup red quinoa, rinsed and drained
2 cups packed fresh basil
¼ cup pine nuts, plus more for serving
¼ cup oil-packed sun-dried tomatoes,
  with 2 tablespoons oil reserved
1 clove garlic

½ teaspoon sea salt
2 to 3 tablespoons extra-virgin
  olive oil
2 cups chopped spinach
1 (15-ounce) can cannellini beans,
  rinsed and drained

In a medium saucepan over high heat, combine the broth and quinoa and bring to a boil. Cover, reduce the heat to low, and simmer for 20 minutes without stirring. Measure 1 cup of the quinoa for use in the salad and save the rest for an easy leftover side dish.

Meanwhile, in a food processor or blender, combine the basil, pine nuts, tomatoes with oil, garlic, and salt. Pulse a few times, then blend while drizzling in the olive oil until thoroughly incorporated.

In a large bowl, combine the quinoa, spinach, and beans and toss with the pesto until well coated. Top with additional pine nuts before serving, if desired.

Spicy Thai Peanut Bowl

1½ cups plus ⅓ cup vegetable broth
1 cup Bhutanese red rice, rinsed
  and drained
3 tablespoons chunky peanut butter
3 tablespoons gluten-free tamari
2 tablespoons rice vinegar
2 teaspoons agave nectar or raw
  honey
2 teaspoons red chili paste

1 teaspoon minced fresh ginger
1 clove garlic, minced
1 cup frozen shelled edamame,
  thawed
2 cups chopped spinach
1 red bell pepper, thinly sliced
1 cooked chicken breast, diced, or
  ½ pound cooked ground turkey
  (optional)

In a medium saucepan over high heat, combine 1½ cups of the broth and the rice and bring to a boil. Cover, reduce the heat to low, and simmer for 20 minutes. Measure 1 cup of the rice for use in the salad and save the rest for an easy leftover side dish.

Meanwhile, in a small bowl, whisk together the remaining ⅓ cup broth, peanut butter, tamari, vinegar, agave, chili paste, ginger, and garlic until thoroughly combined and creamy.

In a large bowl, toss the rice, edamame, spinach, bell pepper, and chicken with the peanut sauce until well coated.

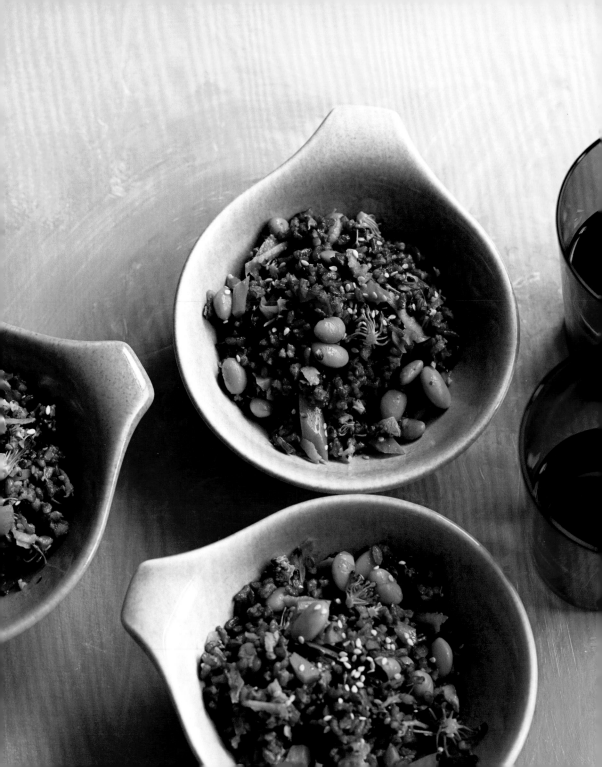

Asian Sesame-Ginger Bowl

1½ cups vegetable broth
1 cup Bhutanese red rice, rinsed and
   drained
¼ cup toasted sesame oil
3 tablespoons rice wine vinegar
2 tablespoons gluten-free tamari
1 tablespoon tahini

½ teaspoon minced fresh ginger
1 head broccoli
1 cup frozen shelled edamame,
   thawed
2 carrots, diced
2 tablespoons sesame seeds

In a medium saucepan over high heat, combine the broth and rice and bring to a boil. Cover, reduce the heat to low, and simmer for 20 minutes. Measure 1 cup of the rice for use in the salad and save the rest for an easy leftover side dish.

Meanwhile, in a small bowl, whisk together the oil, vinegar, tamari, tahini, and ginger.

Chop the broccoli florets into small pieces and shred the stem. In a large bowl, add the broccoli, rice, edamame, and carrots. Drizzle with the dressing, sprinkle with the sesame seeds, and toss until well coated.

BRAIN FOOD FACT

Bhutanese red rice is a great complex carbohydrate that provides fuel for the brain. It's also a good source of magnesium, which has a calming effect on the brain and might be helpful in reducing anxiety.

Massaged Kale and Black-Eyed Peas Bowl

2½ cups mushroom broth

1 cup brown rice

1 bunch kale, stemmed and
coarsely chopped

½ avocado

½ teaspoon sea salt

1 (15-ounce) can black-eyed peas,
rinsed and drained

2 tablespoons extra-virgin olive oil

2 tablespoons balsamic vinegar

In a medium saucepan over high heat, combine the broth and rice and bring to a boil. Cover, reduce the heat to low, and simmer for 45 to 50 minutes, or until the rice is tender. Measure 1 cup of the rice for use in the salad and save the rest for an easy leftover side dish.

In a large bowl, put the kale. Scoop in the avocado and sprinkle with the salt. Using both hands, massage the avocado into the kale. It will start to take on a wilted appearance as it gets tender. Add the rice, black-eyed peas, oil, and vinegar and toss until well combined.

TIME-SAVING TIP

Look for precooked brown rice in the freezer section of your grocery store. It's great to have on hand for an easy side dish and will come in handy for variations of the beans, greens, and grains bowls!

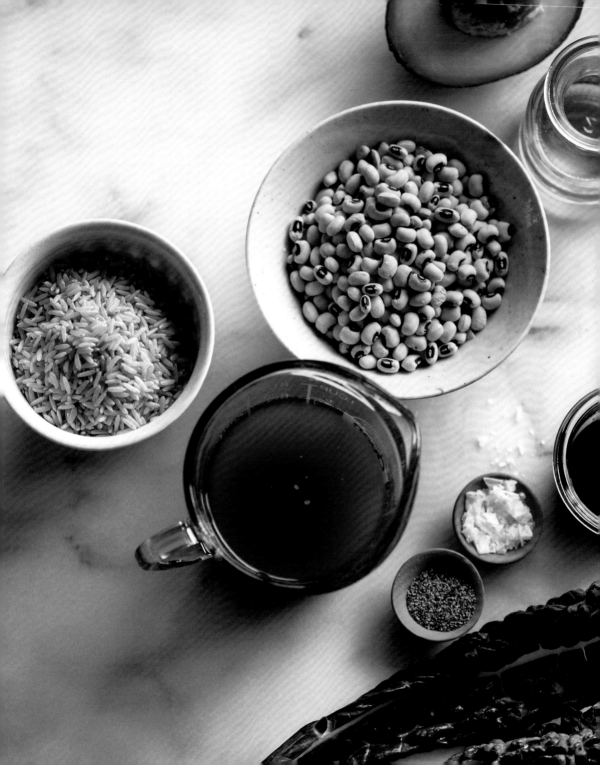

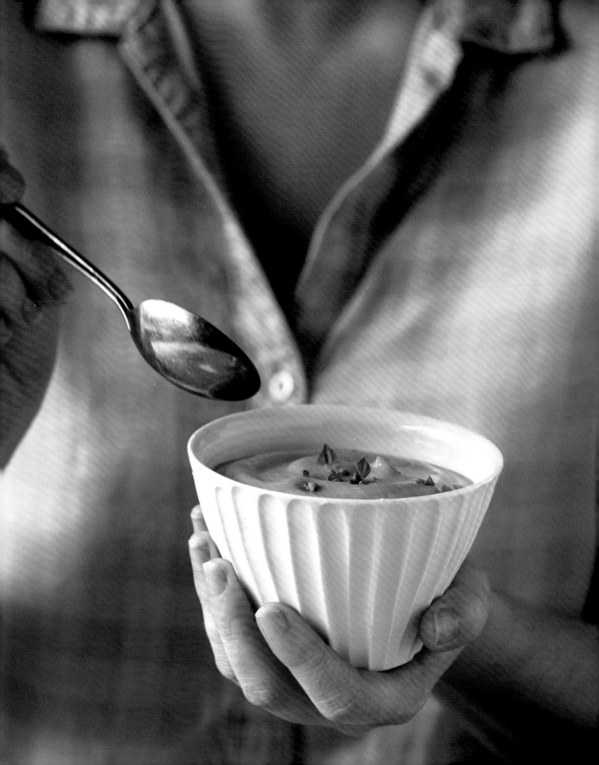

Well-Adjusted Accompaniments

»»««

*Cauliflower is nothing but cabbage
with a college education.*

—MARK TWAIN

>»»«««

>»»«««

Crispy Broccoli and Cauliflower with Cashew Drizzle

I have a confession to make. I don't love broccoli and cauliflower as much as I should. Cruciferous vegetables, as a category, are the hands-down winner for disease-fighting nutrients, so I'm always looking for ways to get more enjoyment out of them. Roasting them at a high temperature until they start to brown and get crispy makes them a lot more exciting. And adding a simple cashew drizzle just makes them downright sexy. The subtle sweetness from the cashews perfectly compliments the saltiness of the seasoned broccoli and cauliflower. No cheese sauce needed!

Makes 4 servings

- 1 small head cauliflower, separated into small florets
- 1 head broccoli, separated into small florets
- 2 tablespoons grapeseed or avocado oil
- 2 tablespoons nutritional yeast
- 1½ teaspoons sea salt, divided
- ½ teaspoon freshly ground black pepper
- ½ teaspoon granulated garlic
- ½ cup raw cashews
- ½ cup water

Preheat the oven to 450 degrees F.

In a large bowl, toss together the cauliflower, broccoli, oil, nutritional yeast, 1 teaspoon of the salt, pepper, and garlic. Spread in a single layer on a large baking sheet and bake for 15 minutes, turning the vegetables halfway through cooking.

Meanwhile, in a food processor, put the cashews and the remaining ½ teaspoon salt and pulse a few times. With the motor running, pour in the water and blend until the consistency resembles a thin, creamy soup.

Transfer the vegetables to plates for serving and drizzle with the cashew mixture.

Sauerkraut Salad with Sautéed Mushrooms

DIFFICULTY METER
● ● ○ ○ ○

If you're reading this recipe, you can count yourself among those whom I consider open minded, and perhaps even adventurous, when it comes to food. My recipe-testing friends had their doubts about this one until they took their first bite. The rich, savory flavor from the sautéed mushrooms paired with the tangy goodness of kraut creates the ultimate umami experience.

Makes 4 servings

4 cups mixed greens
2 tablespoons extra-virgin olive oil
12 shiitake mushrooms, thinly sliced
½ teaspoon sea salt
¼ cup olive oil mayonnaise or
  Vegenaise

2 teaspoons chili sauce
½ teaspoon gluten-free Worcestershire sauce (such as Lea & Perrins)
1 cup sauerkraut

In a large bowl, put the greens.

In a large skillet over medium heat, drizzle the oil and immediately add the mushrooms, stirring until well coated. Sprinkle with the salt and continue to sauté for 4 to 5 minutes, or until the mushrooms are tender and juicy. Transfer to the bowl of greens and toss gently.

Meanwhile, in a small bowl, whisk together the mayonnaise, chili sauce, and Worcestershire.

Add the sauerkraut to the greens and toss with the dressing.

TIME-SAVING TIP

You'll find a recipe to make your own sauerkraut on page 139. If you're not ready for Fermentation 101, you can find good-quality sauerkraut in the refrigerated section of the supermarket. It should be preservative-free and contain no vinegar.

Caprese Salad with Tomato, Basil, and Avocado

The big draw of caprese salad, aside from the simplicity, is the phenomenal flavor and texture combination of basil, tomatoes, and mozzarella. As a person who doesn't tolerate dairy, I had to experiment with other options to replace the mozzarella. Enter avocado and hearts of palm. The avocado gives me that creamy texture that's reminiscent of soft cheese, while the hearts of palm lend a salty, tangy flare. If you can't find hearts of palm, water chestnuts or artichoke hearts are good substitutes. I like to use cherry or grape tomatoes, but you could also arrange the ingredients on sliced tomatoes for a lovely looking hors d'oeuvre.

Makes 6 servings

1 (14-ounce) can hearts of palm, drained and sliced into rounds
1 pint cherry tomatoes
1 avocado, cut into 1-inch pieces
1 cup packed fresh basil, stemmed and torn into bite-size pieces

3 tablespoons extra-virgin olive oil
1 tablespoon balsamic vinegar
½ teaspoon sea salt
Freshly ground black pepper

In a large bowl, combine the hearts of palm, tomatoes, avocado, and basil. Drizzle with the oil and vinegar and toss gently until the ingredients are well coated. Add the salt and season with pepper to taste. Serve immediately.

Smoky Yam and Kale Salad

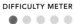

One of my favorite vegan restaurants uses smoked paprika liberally, and I always feel like it gives vegetables and legumes a deeper, richer flavor that's so satisfying and really makes you forget you're not eating meat. The paprika pairs nicely with turmeric too, so this can be a nice go-to spice combo when you're looking for ways to incorporate more turmeric. You can use any type of kale you like in this recipe, but I prefer leafy kale for how it crisps up in the oven.

Makes 4 servings

- 2 unpeeled garnet yams, cut into ½-inch cubes
- 3 tablespoons avocado oil or sunflower oil, divided
- 1 bunch curly kale (such as red Russian), stemmed and chopped
- 1 tablespoon ground turmeric
- 1½ teaspoons smoked paprika
- 1 teaspoon sea salt
- 1 tablespoon balsamic vinegar

Preheat the oven to 425 degrees F.

In a large bowl, toss the yams with 2 tablespoons of the oil. In a separate bowl, toss the kale with the remaining 1 tablespoon oil.

In a small bowl, combine the turmeric, paprika, and salt. Sprinkle half of the mixture over the yams and half over the kale. Toss both until well coated. Set the kale aside, spread the yams in a single layer on a large baking sheet, and bake for 20 minutes, stirring halfway through cooking. Spread the kale over the yams and bake for another 7 minutes.

Transfer the yams and kale back to a large bowl and toss with the vinegar. This salad can be served warm or cold.

Spinach-Arugula Salad with Curried Pumpkin Seeds

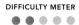

All it takes to make salads more interesting is some arugula and a little imagination. Spinach is a nutritional powerhouse but can be, well, kinda boring. So jazzing it up with some spicy greens, like arugula, and adding some crunch with kick, like curried pumpkin seeds, really make this salad come to life.

Makes 4 servings

¼ cup extra-virgin olive oil
1 tablespoon sherry vinegar
1 teaspoon raw honey
¼ teaspoon sea salt
2 cups spinach

1 cup arugula
1 red bell pepper, thinly sliced
½ cup shredded carrots
½ cup Sassy Punks (page 62)

In a small bowl, whisk together the oil, vinegar, honey, and salt.

In a large bowl, combine the spinach, arugula, bell pepper, and carrots. Drizzle with the dressing and toss until the ingredients are well coated. Divide among four salad plates, top each with 2 tablespoons Sassy Punks, and serve.

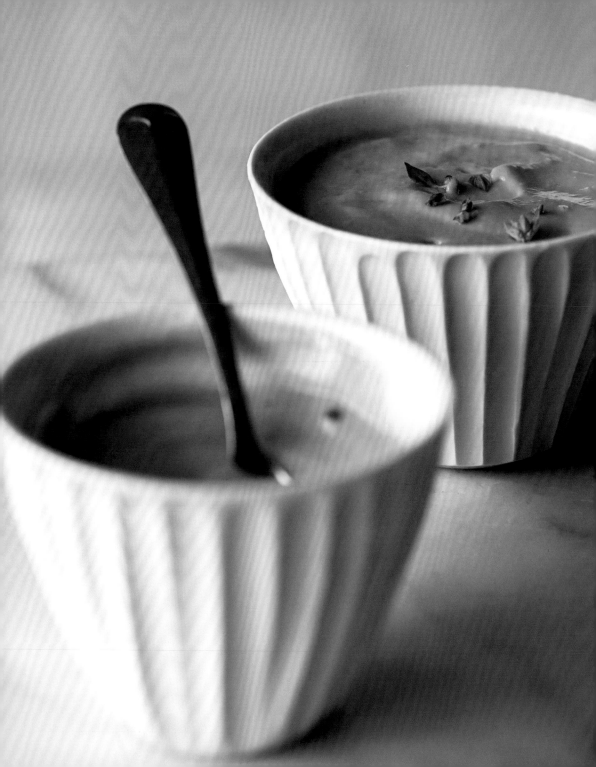

Blend-and-Heat Soups

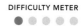

My blender soup recipes were born out of a recurring request from clients for more ideas for portable meals. Those busy parents who are racing out the door to shuttle kids to and from their many activities enjoy having something nourishing that they can throw in a travel mug and take on the road. While I prefer that people sit and savor their meals, I'm willing to concede that sipping on a veggie-packed soup beats the alternatives of not eating or grabbing a protein bar out of desperation.

Makes 4 servings (each option)

Calm, Cool Basil-Avocado Soup

2 ripe avocados, halved
½ English cucumber, peeled and seeded
5 to 7 fresh basil leaves
1½ cups vegetable broth

1 cup water
2 teaspoons freshly squeezed lime juice
1 teaspoon ume plum vinegar
1 teaspoon sea salt

Scoop the avocados into a powerful blender or food processor and add all the remaining ingredients. Blend until smooth, adding more water or broth as desired. Serve cold.

BRAIN FOOD FACT

Avocados provide nearly twenty essential nutrients and are a rich source of folate and B_6, which are essential for serotonin and dopamine production.

Spicy Tortilla Soup with Black Beans

2 cups warm water
2 Roma tomatoes
1 carrot
½ avocado
1 shallot
⅓ cup fire-roasted peppers

2 tablespoons fresh cilantro
1 teaspoon sea salt
1 teaspoon chili powder
¾ teaspoon granulated garlic
¾ cup black beans
Tortilla chips, for garnish (optional)

In a powerful blender or food processor, combine the water, tomatoes, carrot, avocado, shallot, peppers, cilantro, salt, chili powder, and garlic and blend until smooth. Transfer the soup to a saucepan or microwave-safe dish, stir in the beans, and heat through. Serve warm, garnished with the tortilla chips.

Creamy Carrot-Ginger Soup

1½ cups vegetable broth
½ cup water
3 medium carrots
⅓ cup silken tofu
¼ cup frozen butternut squash,
    thawed

1 shallot, halved
2 cloves garlic
2 teaspoons minced fresh ginger
1 teaspoon sea salt

In a powerful blender or food processor, combine all the ingredients and blend until smooth. Transfer the soup to a saucepan or microwave-safe dish and heat through. Serve warm.

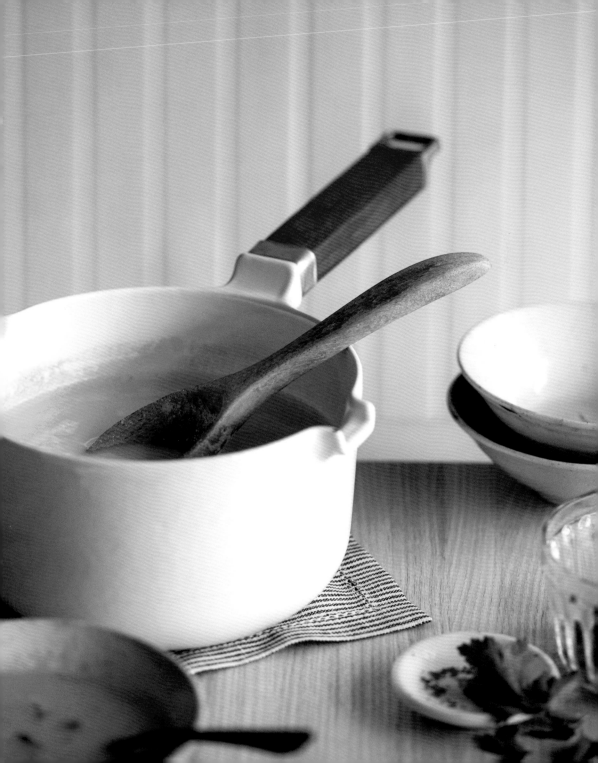

Silky Sunchoke and Celeriac Soup

When I teach cooking classes, I like to feature some of the ugly ducklings of the vegetable kingdom and transform them into something irresistible. Sunchokes and celeriac are a couple of those not-so-cute, somewhat-intimidating kinds of vegetables. I describe celeriac as celery on steroids. It's bold in flavor but has a more potato-like texture, so there are no stringy fibers to contend with. The sunchokes resemble overgrown ginger but have a nice nutty flavor with a hint of artichoke.

Makes 6 servings

4 sunchokes (Jerusalem artichokes), well scrubbed and cut into 1-inch chunks

1 medium celeriac (celery root), peeled and cut into 1-inch chunks

3 cups mushroom broth

1 tablespoon dried Italian herbs

2 teaspoons sea salt

1 teaspoon freshly ground black pepper

½ teaspoon freshly grated lemon zest

Place the sunchokes and celeriac in a steamer basket set over simmering water and steam until tender, about 15 minutes. Transfer the vegetables to a food processor. Add the broth, Italian herbs, salt, pepper, and lemon zest and puree until smooth. Transfer the soup to a medium saucepan over medium-low heat and serve warm.

Roasted Beets with Crushed Macadamia Nuts

I challenge you to use this recipe on any friend or family member who claims to dislike beets. Roasted beets are such a different culinary experience than steamed ones; they're sweeter, less earthy, and have a much better texture. The ume plum vinegar adds a touch of umami that plays well on the palate and masks any remaining earthiness. And as if that isn't enough, top it all off with the most perfect, exotic nut that ever lived. How can anyone resist?

Makes 4 servings

6 beets, scrubbed, trimmed, and
    chopped into 1-inch pieces
1 tablespoon sunflower oil
2 teaspoons coarse sea salt

2 teaspoons ume plum vinegar
¼ cup roasted macadamia nuts,
    coarsely chopped

Preheat the oven to 375 degrees F.

In a medium bowl, toss the beets with the oil and salt until well coated. Spread the beets in a single layer on a baking sheet and roast for about 25 minutes, or until the beets are tender.

Drizzle with the vinegar and toss to coat. Divide the beets among four plates and top each with about 1 tablespoon of the macadamia nuts.

BRAIN FOOD FACT

Beets contain some very unique phytonutrients that have been shown to inhibit COX-1 and COX-2 enzymes. These enzymes send signals that trigger inflammation. In this way beets operate similarly to nonsteroidal anti-inflammatory drugs but without the unwanted side effects.

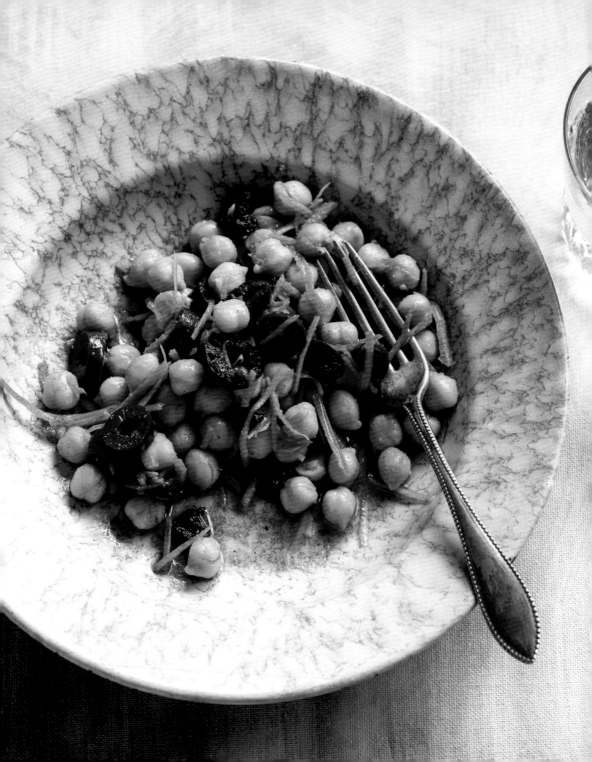

Moroccan Chickpea Salad

DIFFICULTY METER
● ● ● ● ●

This recipe was inspired by a Turkish chickpea dish that's featured in the PCC deli. That's what proved to me that you can successfully combine dried fruit and olives to produce a salty-sweet combo that's positively mouthwatering. This is one of those salads that actually gets better as it sits and marinates for a couple days. I like to make this one the night before I want to serve it. It's great to take to work for lunch or as a snack, and it also does well in a cooler for camping trips.

Makes 4 servings

¼ cup extra-virgin olive oil
2 tablespoons sherry vinegar
1 clove garlic, minced
1 teaspoon ground cumin
½ teaspoon ground ginger
½ teaspoon sea salt
½ teaspoon ground white pepper
½ teaspoon ground cinnamon

¼ teaspoon ground coriander
1 (15-ounce) can chickpeas, rinsed
    and drained
½ cup shredded carrots
½ cup pitted kalamata olives,
    chopped
¼ cup raisins

In a small bowl, whisk together the oil, vinegar, garlic, cumin, ginger, salt, pepper, cinnamon, and coriander.

In a large bowl, combine the chickpeas, carrots, olives, and raisins. Drizzle with the dressing and toss until well coated.

BRAIN FOOD FACT

Chickpeas are a great source of insoluble fiber, which feeds the good bacteria in the gut and may even improve your gut-brain communication. Not to mention that beans help balance blood sugar to stabilize mood and energy.

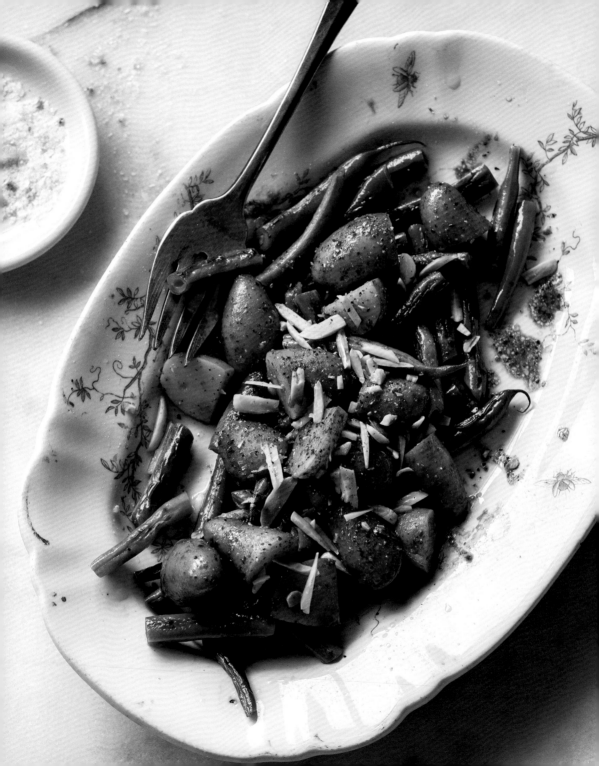

Potato and Roasted Green Bean Salad with Slivered Almonds

I've always been a sucker for a good potato salad but I'm not generally a fan of heavy mayo. This is a much lighter take on a potato salad, and I even invited green beans to the party. After being a victim of the canned versions as a child, I fell in love with green beans much later in life once I discovered roasting is the ticket. This is also a small attempt to get potatoes, which have gotten an undeserved bad rap, back on the plate. In Dr. DesMaisons's famous book *Potatoes Not Prozac*, she recommends eating a potato three hours after dinner to help boost serotonin levels. One cup of this salad might just be the perfect mood-enhancing bedtime snack!

Makes 6 servings

12 to 15 fingerling potatoes
3 cups green beans, cut into
   1-inch pieces
4 tablespoons extra-virgin olive
   oil, divided
1 teaspoon kosher salt
2 tablespoons balsamic vinegar

1 tablespoon Dijon or
   stone-ground mustard
1 teaspoon sea salt
½ teaspoon freshly ground
   black pepper
¼ cup slivered almonds

Preheat the oven to 375 degrees F.

In large saucepan, put the potatoes and cover with water. Bring the water to a boil, reduce the heat to medium, and simmer for about 10 minutes, or until the potatoes are tender. Drain, rinse under cold water, and refrigerate until cool.

In a medium bowl, toss the green beans with 1 tablespoon of the oil and kosher salt. Spread them in a single layer on a baking sheet and roast for 15 minutes, or until the green beans start to brown.

Meanwhile, in a small bowl, whisk together the remaining 3 tablespoons oil, the vinegar, and mustard.

CONTINUED

Slice the cooled potatoes into quarters and put them in a large bowl. Add the green beans, drizzle with the vinaigrette, and toss gently until the vegetables are well coated. Season with the salt and pepper.

In a small dry pan over medium heat, lightly toast the almonds, stirring frequently, for about 3 minutes, or until they begin to brown and become fragrant. Sprinkle over the salad and serve.

BRAIN FOOD FACT

Potatoes are a very good source of vitamin B_6, which is necessary for the production of all the key neurotransmitters like dopamine, serotonin, melatonin, norepinephrine, and GABA. Think of potatoes as powerful gut-brain communication builder.

Sesame-Ginger Slaw with Jicama

When you think of slaw, a mayonnaise-based dressing might come to mind. But this is not your granny's coleslaw. The fresh, zesty sesame-ginger dressing in this version brightens up the cabbage, and the jicama gives it a sweet, light crunch. This is my go-to slaw when I make fish tacos. It also gets better as it marinates in the fridge for a couple days, so it's the perfect side dish to make on a Sunday and enjoy through the first part of the week.

Makes 4 servings

½ small head green cabbage
½ small head purple cabbage
1 jicama, cut roughly into strips
3 tablespoons brown rice vinegar

2 tablespoons toasted sesame oil
1 tablespoon flaxseed oil
1 tablespoon raw honey
1 teaspoon minced fresh ginger

In a food processor fitted with the shredding attachment, shred the cabbages and jicama. Alternatively, you can thinly slice the cabbages with a knife and shred the jicama with a grater. Transfer the vegetables to a large bowl.

In a small bowl, whisk together the vinegar, oils, honey, and ginger. Drizzle over the slaw and toss until well coated.

BRAIN FOOD FACT

Jicama features a unique form of fiber called inulin, which is a beneficial prebiotic food that stimulates the activity of healthy bacteria growth in the gut.

Fennel and Spring Onion Salad
with Blood Orange Vinaigrette

If you're bored to tears by the standard green salad, I've got the cure. The key to making a salad more interesting is adding different textures, inviting new and exciting flavors to the party, and tossing it all with a perfectly balanced dressing. Fennel is known for its anise-type flavor, so slicing it thinly prevents it from being overpowering and adds just the right amount of intrigue. The zing from the onion and the sweetness from the bell pepper play well with the fennel, and the sweet-tart blood orange dressing is a unique departure from your usual vinaigrette.

Makes 4 servings

Juice from 2 blood oranges, or juice from 1 navel orange if blood oranges aren't available (about 3 to 4 tablespoons)
¼ cup extra-virgin olive oil
1 tablespoon rice vinegar
½ teaspoon sea salt
4 cups mixed greens
1 large fennel bulb, stemmed and trimmed, thinly sliced
1 spring or red onion, thinly sliced
1 red bell pepper, thinly sliced

In a small bowl, whisk together the juice, oil, vinegar, and salt.

In a large bowl, combine the greens, fennel, onion, and bell pepper. Drizzle with the vinaigrette and toss until well coated.

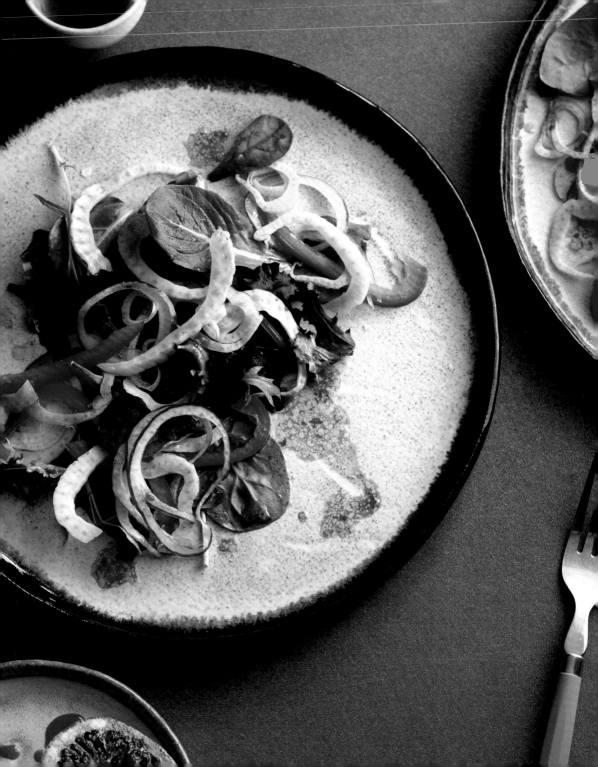

Creamy Broccoli Soup with
Fire-Roasted Peppers

Cream-based soups were something I really missed when I had to omit dairy from my diet. Strategically using potatoes to emulate creaminess is a brilliant way to sidestep dairy and boost nutritional value in this recipe. The sautéed leeks add a buttery note and the nutritional yeast is like a whisper of Parmesan. This soup is the perfect starter for just about any meal and a delicious accompaniment to most fish dishes.

Makes 4 servings

2 medium Yukon gold potatoes, peeled and chopped into 2-inch chunks
1 head broccoli
1 tablespoon extra-virgin olive oil
1 medium leek, white and light-green parts only, rinsed well and sliced into half moons
1 stalk celery, sliced

2 cloves garlic, minced
½ cup unsweetened almond or cashew milk
3 tablespoons nutritional yeast
1 tablespoon gluten-free tamari
1 teaspoon sea salt
½ teaspoon ground white pepper
½ cup sliced fire-roasted peppers
Chili oil, for drizzling

In a large saucepan or stockpot, put the potatoes. Trim the broccoli stem, chop it into 2-inch chunks, and add it to the pan. Cover the vegetables with water by about 2 inches. Set the pan over high heat and bring the water to a boil. Reduce the heat to medium and cook for 10 minutes. Break off the broccoli florets and add them to the pot. Cover and cook for 2 minutes, or until the vegetables are easily pieced with a fork. Strain and reserve the cooking water. Transfer the vegetables to a food processor. (Alternatively, you can use an immersion blender to puree the soup.)

Meanwhile, heat the olive oil in a sauté pan over medium heat. Add the leeks, celery, and garlic and sauté for 5 to 7 minutes, or until the leeks start to brown on the edges and the celery begins to soften. Transfer the vegetables to the food processor (or the saucepan, if using an immersion blender). Add the almond milk, nutritional yeast, tamari, salt, and pepper. Blend the soup, slowly pouring in the reserved cooking water until it reaches your desired consistency. Return the soup to the saucepan and reheat.

Ladle the soup into four bowls, top each with 2 tablespoons fire-roasted peppers, drizzle with chili oil, and serve.

BRAIN FOOD FACT

Broccoli has an unusually strong combination of beta-carotene and vitamin K, both of which have powerful anti-inflammatory powers.

Broccoli is a rich source of a flavonoid called kaempferol, which defends the body against allergens and decreases the inflammatory response. Broccoli is also loaded with vitamin K, which is a powerful anti-inflammatory nutrient and also helps aid in the absorption of vitamin D.

Braised Kale with Roasted Garlic–Tahini Dressing

DIFFICULTY METER
● ● ● ◌ ◌

To braise something simply means to sauté it in a fat or oil and then stew it in a small amount of liquid. Braising some of the heartier greens, like kale, helps break them down and makes them much more enjoyable to eat (and easier to digest). Tossing the braised kale with the garlic-tahini dressing creates the perfect marriage of flavors and eliminates any bitter notes from the greens. I like to pile this in the middle of a plate and plop a nice piece of grilled whitefish right on top. If I don't have fish to grill, I've also been known to mash in some canned sardines for a big omega-3 boost.

Makes 4 servings

1 head garlic
4 tablespoons plus ½ teaspoon extra-virgin olive oil, divided
¼ cup water
¼ cup tahini
1 tablespoon balsamic vinegar
1½ teaspoons sea salt, divided

1 shallot, diced
1 cup sliced shiitake mushrooms
1 bunch Tuscan kale, stemmed and chopped
1 bunch curly kale (such as red Russian), stemmed and chopped
¼ cup mushroom broth

Preheat the oven to 370 degrees F.

Slice the top off the head of garlic just enough to expose the cloves. Drizzle with ½ teaspoon of the oil, wrap in foil, and roast for 45 minutes. Allow the garlic to cool slightly before squeezing the cloves into a small bowl. Add the water, tahini, vinegar, 2 tablespoons of the oil, and ½ teaspoon of the salt and whisk until smooth.

Heat the remaining 2 tablespoons oil in a large sauté pan over medium heat. Add the shallot and cook for 2 minutes. Add the mushrooms and remaining 1 teaspoon salt and sauté for 5 minutes. Add all of the kale and sauté until it begins to wilt, about 3 minutes. Reduce the heat to low, pour in the broth, cover, and simmer for 5 minutes. Remove the pan from the heat.

Drizzle the kale with the dressing, toss well, and serve warm.

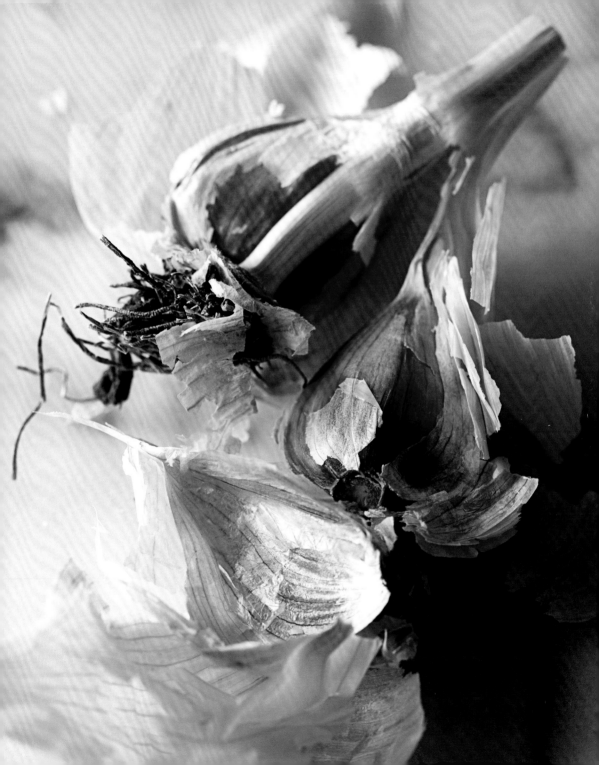

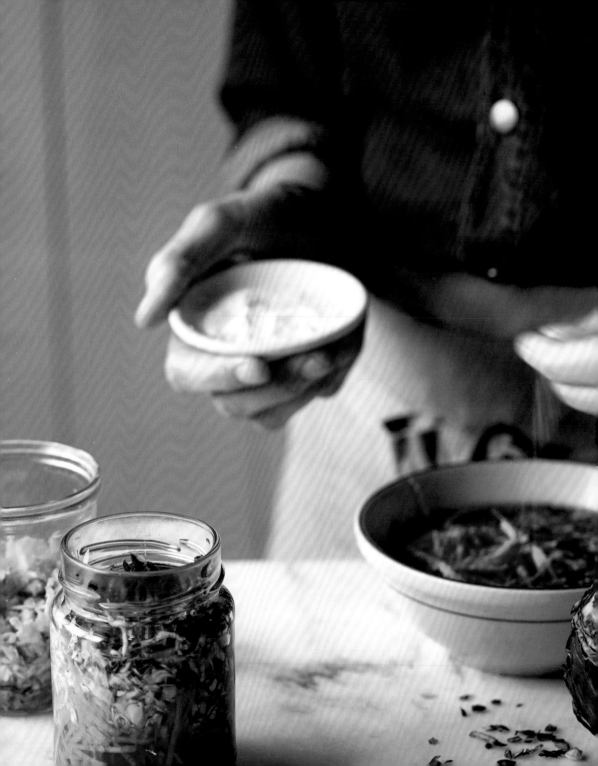

Gut-Harmonizing Helpers

»»««

To ferment your own food is to lodge a small but eloquent protest—on behalf of the senses and microbes—against the homogenization of flavors and food experiences.

—MICHAEL POLLAN

»»««

FABULOUSLY FERMENTED KRAUT THREE WAYS   139
Golden Curry Kraut with Beets and Turmeric

Carrot-Ginger Kraut

Cruciferous Kraut

CLEVERLY CULTURED FOODS   143
Soy Yogurt

Blue-Raspberry Kefir

Raspberry Yogurt Swirl

»»««

Fabulously Fermented Kraut
Three Ways

All of this attention to the state of our microbiome has led to lots of innovation in the world of fermentation. There are now numerous options for krauts and kimchis available in the supermarket, but if you're going to eat fermented foods on a regular basis, this can quickly become spendy. Thankfully, it's extremely simple and very gratifying to ferment your own foods right at home.

I'm providing some very basic guidelines (adapted from *Fermented Vegetables* by Kirsten K. Shockey and Christopher Shockey) and a few recipe options to pique your interest, but there are lots of great resources available that can give you more comprehensive information. I know that I, for one, resisted the idea of home-fermentation because of my fears about food safety. But lacto-fermentation is a method of preservation that has been used since the beginning of time. Not only is it safe and effective, it produces living food that's teeming with beneficial bacteria that aid in digestion, bolster the immune system, reduce inflammation, and improve gut-brain communication. So I conquered my fermentation phobia and thoroughly enjoy my gourmet homemade krauts—and my pocketbook thanks me too.

Makes about 2 quarts (each option)

GOLDEN CURRY KRAUT WITH BEETS AND TURMERIC

2 pounds green cabbage, shredded

2 medium golden beets, trimmed, scrubbed, and shredded

1-inch piece turmeric, peeled and shredded

1 tablespoon Himalayan crystal salt or sea salt

1 teaspoon whole cumin seeds

CARROT-GINGER KRAUT

1 pound green cabbage, shredded

1 pound purple cabbage, shredded

½ pound carrots, shredded

1-inch piece fresh ginger, peeled and shredded

1 tablespoon Himalayan crystal salt or sea salt

1 teaspoon whole caraway seeds

CONTINUED

CRUCIFEROUS KRAUT

2 pounds green cabbage, shredded
1 pound cauliflower, florets
   thinly sliced
1 tablespoon Himalayan crystal salt
   or sea salt
1 tablespoon minced fresh dill

Rinse the vegetables in cool water and place in a large bowl.

Add ½ tablespoon of the salt and massage it into the vegetables with your hands. Let the vegetables stand for 30 to 45 minutes to start creating a brine. Hand-toss the vegetables with the remaining ½ tablespoon salt—add the salt gradually and taste along the way to ensure the vegetables are well seasoned and not overly salty. (No need to add all of the remaining salt if you're satisfied with less.) Stir in herbs and spices.

Transfer the vegetables to a crock or half-gallon mason jar and press down with your fist or a tamper to release more brine. Leave 2 to 3 inches of headspace in the container and cover the vegetables with one or two whole cabbage leaves to prevent floaters above the liquid line. Top with a secondary follower and a weight (this can be a plate topped with a sealed, water-filled jar for a crock, or a water-filled ziplock freezer bag for a mason jar).

Place the crock on a rimmed baking sheet out of direct sunlight in a cool area (between 55 and 75 degrees F). If using a jar, cover it with a kitchen towel to protect the contents from light.

Allow to ferment for 4 to 6 weeks, tamping the vegetables down as needed to make sure they are always submerged. Skim off any visible scum or mold and discard.

Do a taste check at the 4-week mark; the kraut should be pleasingly sour, and the other vegetables should have softened but still retained a bit of crunch. If the vegetables taste salty and not sour enough or they are still too crispy, allow to ferment for another week before tasting again.

Transfer the kraut to smaller jars with lids and store in the refrigerator for up to 2 months.

These fermented recipes are ranked at a medium difficulty level because they require some ongoing monitoring and management. Prepping and combining the ingredients is quick and simple, and the whole process will become easier to manage with practice.

FURTHER READING

Here are a few resources for learning more about fermentation:

» *Nourishing Traditions* by Sally Fallon

» *Wild Fermentation* by Sandor Ellix Katz

» *Fermented Vegetables* by Kirsten K. Shockey and Christopher Shockey

TOOLS OF THE TRADE

» Ceramic crock or large mason jars for smaller batches

» Followers (these are weights that keep the vegetables submerged in brine)

» Lid with airlock (optional but makes it easier to manage the volatility of CO_2 release)

» FARMcurious.com has some great fermentation starter kits

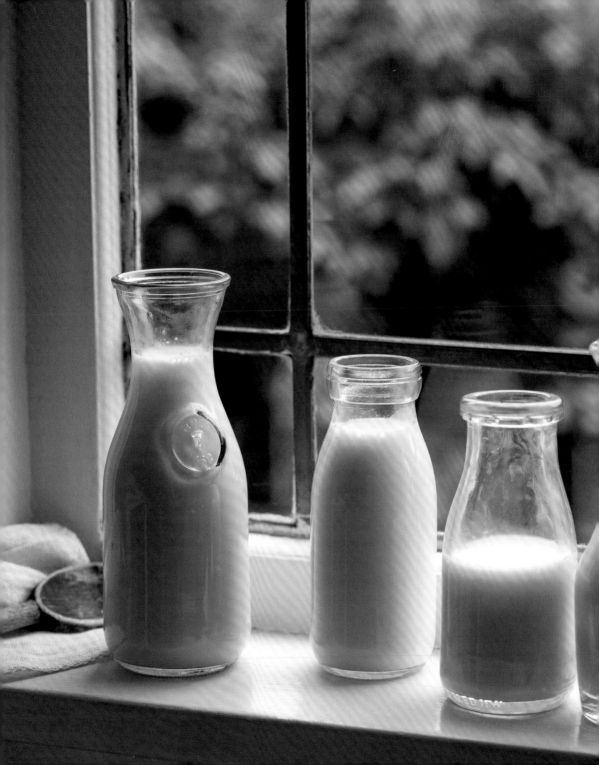

Cleverly Cultured Foods

Cultured cow's milk, coconut milk, or soymilk is a tasty way to bring more beneficial bacteria into your milieu, and it's faster and even easier than fermenting foods. The *Lactobacillus acidophilus* that thrives in yogurt and kefir is what is commonly sold in supplemental form as probiotics, and it has been associated with improved digestion, reduced inflammation, and a reduction in depressive symptoms. Kefir grains look like little pieces of cauliflower and can be purchased at your local health food store or ordered online.

Makes 1 quart (each option)

Soy Yogurt

1 quart organic plain unsweetened soymilk (I like WestSoy or Eden Soy)

1 tablespoon plain unsweetened soy yogurt that contains live cultures

In a medium saucepan over medium heat, bring the soy milk to 180 degrees F (use a thermometer). Stir frequently, scraping the bottom of the pan to avoid scorching the milk.

Cool the milk to exactly 110 degrees F (don't let it drop below that temperature) and immediately mix in the live-culture yogurt.

Transfer the mixture to a quart jar. Cover the jar and place it in an insulated cooler or a warm spot in the kitchen. Let the mixture sit for 8 to 12 hours without disturbing it.

Taste the yogurt after 8 hours—it should be thick with some tang to it. If it's still not tangy enough, allow to sit for another couple hours before tasting again. Remove at least 1 tablespoon of the yogurt to use as a starter for the next batch and store it in a covered container for up to 1 week in the refrigerator or up to 3 weeks in the freezer.

Serve the yogurt, or store in the refrigerator for up to 2 weeks. (Note: It will safely keep in the refrigerator for up to 1 month, but it may start to taste sour.)

Blue-Raspberry Kefir

1 tablespoon kefir grains
1 quart organic whole milk
½ cup fresh or frozen blueberries,
thawed

½ cup fresh or frozen raspberries,
thawed
1 tablespoon raw honey

In a large glass jar, put the kefir grains and fill with the milk. Cover with a clean cloth and place on the counter. Let the mixture sit for 1 to 2 days, stirring periodically with a non-metal spoon. When the mixture is thick, carefully strain out the kefir grains with a plastic strainer. Place the grains in a clean jar and repeat to maintain rotating jars of kefir. The grains can be stored in water in a sealed glass jar in the refrigerator for up to 2 weeks when not in use.

Combine the blueberries, raspberries, and honey in a blender and pulse several times. Stir the mixture into the kefir and serve, or store in the refrigerator for up to 2 weeks.

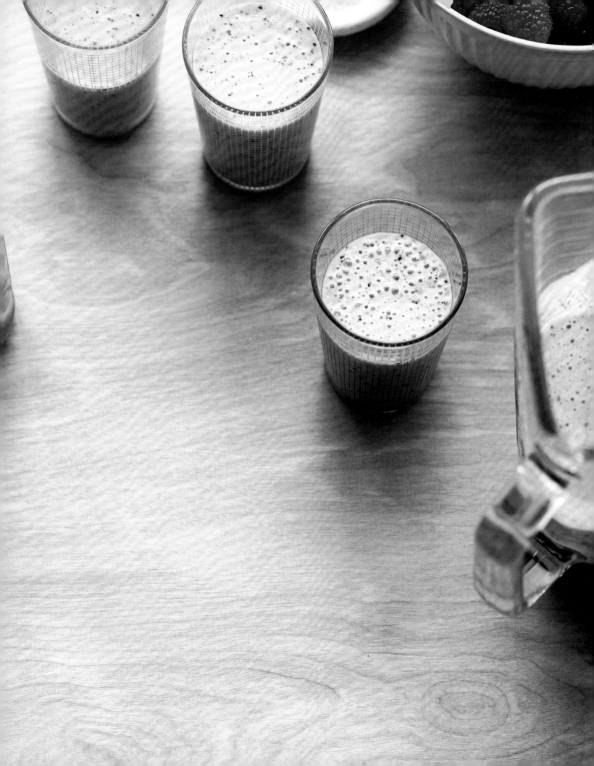

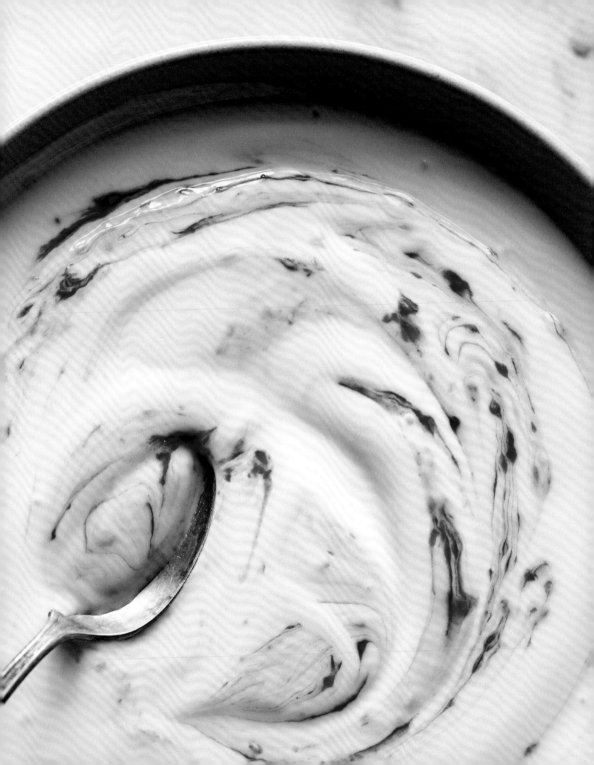

Raspberry Yogurt Swirl

1 quart organic whole milk
1 tablespoon plain unsweetened
   yogurt containing live cultures

1 cup fresh or frozen raspberries,
   thawed
1 tablespoon raw honey

In a medium saucepan over medium heat, bring the milk to 180 degrees F (use a thermometer). Stir frequently, scraping the bottom of the pan to avoid scorching the milk.

Cool the milk to exactly 110 degrees F (don't let it drop below that temperature) and immediately mix in the live-culture yogurt.

Transfer the mixture to a quart jar. Cover the jar and place it in an insulated cooler or a warm spot in the kitchen. Let the mixture sit for 8 to 12 hours without disturbing it.

Taste the yogurt after 8 hours—it should be thick with some tang to it. If it's still not tangy enough, allow it to sit for another couple hours before tasting again. Remove at least 1 tablespoon of the yogurt to use as a starter for the next batch, and store it in a covered container for up to 1 week in the refrigerator or up to 3 weeks in the freezer.

In a blender, combine the raspberries and honey and pulse several times. Stir the mixture into the yogurt and serve, or store in the refrigerator for up to 2 weeks. (Note: It will safely keep in the refrigerator for up to 1 month, but it may start to taste sour.)

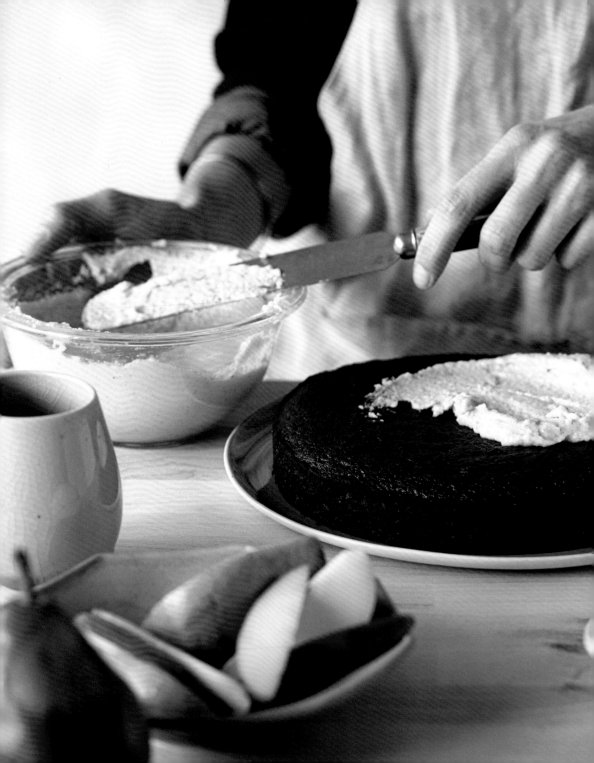

Tantalizing Treats

》》《《

All you need is love. But a little chocolate now and then doesn't hurt.

—CHARLES M. SCHULZ

»»««

»»««

Raw Coconut Fudge Brownies

If you're a chocolate fan, you're going to love the ease and instant gratification of this dessert. There's no waiting around for it to bake—just blend it and press into a pan. You can eat it immediately, though it's best if you let it set up in the refrigerator for a couple hours. The raw coconut butter in this recipe is delicious on its own. Note that coconut *butter* is not the same as coconut *oil*: coconut butter is made from the coconut meat. It's rich and creamy and plays well with cocoa and dates.

Makes 12 brownies

1 cup raw walnuts	¼ cup raw coconut butter
1 cup Medjool dates, pitted	1 vanilla bean
¼ cup unsweetened cocoa powder	2 teaspoons raw agave nectar

In a food processor, combine the walnuts, dates, cocoa, and coconut butter. Use a paring knife to slice the vanilla bean lengthwise down the center. Open the bean to expose the paste-like seeds and use the back of the knife to gently scrape them out of the pod. Add the seeds and agave to the food processor and blend until the mixture resembles a sticky dough.

Transfer the dough into a 9-inch square baking dish and press down firmly with a wooden spoon. Refrigerate for 1 to 2 hours to make it easier to cut the brownies into squares.

Raspberry Chia Pudding

When I want a quick post-dinner treat, my go-to is often some variation of chia pudding. I can make one serving to satisfy my sweet tooth and I absolutely love the tapioca-like texture. I put this together while I'm doing my dinner dishes, then stick it in the refrigerator to gel until I'm ready for my snack. You can use any berry in this recipe, but raspberries lend a tart-sweet flavor and also carry some powerful phytonutrients that might just have mood-altering effects. This recipe can easily be doubled or quadrupled to feed everyone.

Makes 1 serving

½ cup fresh raspberries
2 teaspoons raw honey

¼ cup full-fat, unsweetened coconut
   milk (I use Aroy-D)
2 tablespoons chia seeds

In a small bowl, mash the raspberries with the honey. Stir in the coconut milk and chia seeds. Cover and refrigerate for at least 30 minutes or up to 4 days. The mixture will continue to thicken as it sits, so you may need to add more liquid to get to your desired texture, similar to tapioca pudding.

BRAIN FOOD FACT

The ellagic acid in raspberries appears to block reuptake of serotonin, leaving more of this mood-boosting neurotransmitter for your brain to use.

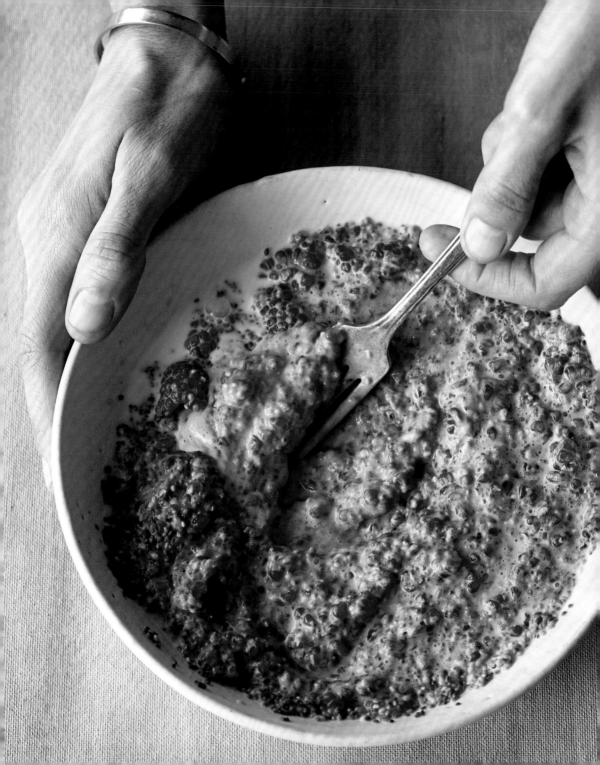

Banana-Almond Mookies

What's a mookie, you ask? A cross between a muffin and cookie, of course! The first time I made these little gems, I pulled them out of the oven and handed one to a friend while describing them as flat muffins. These could actually qualify as a breakfast cookie too. This is one of the easiest baked treats I've ever created.

Makes 8 mookies

1 cup almond flour
¼ cup coconut palm sugar
1 teaspoon ground cinnamon

1 small very ripe banana
1 large egg

Preheat the oven to 325 degrees F.

Sift the flour into a large mixing bowl. Whisk in the coconut sugar and cinnamon. In a small bowl, mash the banana with a fork and whisk in the egg. Fold the banana mixture into the dry ingredients and mix until well combined.

Use a large spoon to scoop the mookie mixture onto the baking sheet in 2-inch rounds. Bake for 15 minutes, or until a toothpick inserted into the center comes out clean. Allow the mookies to cool slightly before serving.

Chocolate Pear Torte

I first made this torte for a cooking class on healthy hormone balance because pears are such a fantastic fruit for stabilizing blood sugar—and putting pears and chocolate together just made sense. What I hadn't expected was how beautiful this dessert would look and how satisfying a small slice can be. One little nibble will promptly make you forget that you're eating a "healthy" dessert.

Makes one 9-inch torte

Coconut oil, for greasing
2 cups almond flour
¼ cup unsweetened cocoa powder
½ teaspoon baking soda
½ teaspoon sea salt
1 cup agave nectar
2 large eggs
1 teaspoon vanilla extract

2 cups raw cashews
½ cup coconut cream
2 tablespoons pure maple syrup
1 vanilla bean
¾ cup water
2 pears, thinly sliced
2 teaspoons ground cinnamon

Preheat the oven to 350 degrees F. Grease a 9-inch springform pan with about 1 teaspoon coconut oil.

In a large bowl, combine the flour, cocoa, baking soda, and salt. In a medium bowl, whisk together the agave, eggs, and vanilla. Stir the wet ingredients into the dry mixture until thoroughly combined. Scoop the batter into the prepared pan and smooth the top.

Bake for 35 to 40 minutes, or until a toothpick inserted into the center of the cake comes out clean. Set aside to cool.

CONTINUED

Meanwhile, in a food processor, combine the cashews, coconut cream, and maple syrup. Use a paring knife to slice the vanilla bean lengthwise down the center. Open the bean to expose the paste-like seeds, use the back of the knife to gently scrape them out of the pod, and add them to the food processor. With the motor running, gradually add the water until the mixture is the consistency of a thick nut butter.

Spread the cashew cream over the cake, pushing it all the way to the sides of the pan. Arrange the pear slices in a circular pattern over the top, then sprinkle with the cinnamon. Remove the springform ring, slice the cake, and serve.

BRAIN FOOD FACT

Researchers have isolated over a dozen phytonutrients in pears that appear to inhibit inflammation and protect the immune system.

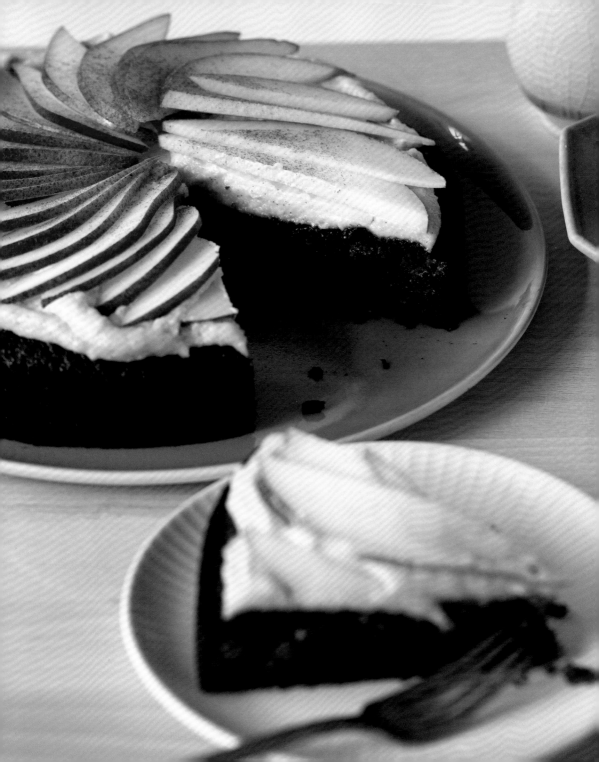

Pumpkin-Coconut Custard
with Walnut-Date Crumble

When my seven-year-old niece made a special request to have this dessert as her birthday treat, I knew I was onto something. I'm a big fan of making single-serving desserts in ramekins. It makes guests (and nieces) feel special when they get their own personal dessert, but it's also good portion practice for those of us who have a little less self-control. The custard, with or without the crumble, actually makes a delicious breakfast when mixed with about ½ cup cooked oatmeal. Now that's the way to make oatmeal considerably more appealing!

Makes 6 servings

FOR THE CUSTARD
2 large eggs
1 (15-ounce) can pumpkin puree
1 cup full-fat, unsweetened
    coconut milk
⅓ cup agave nectar or pure
    maple syrup
2 teaspoons ground cinnamon
½ teaspoon ground ginger
½ teaspoon ground nutmeg
½ teaspoon sea salt
¼ teaspoon ground allspice

FOR THE CRUMBLE
2 cups walnuts
5 Medjool dates, pitted
2 teaspoons ground cinnamon
⅛ teaspoon sea salt

To make the custard, preheat the oven to 375 degrees F. Place six 4-inch ramekins on a baking sheet.

In a large bowl, beat the eggs, then whisk in the pumpkin puree, coconut milk, agave, cinnamon, ginger, nutmeg, salt, and allspice until well combined. Divide the mixture evenly among the ramekins, leaving about 1 inch of space above the batter.

Bake for 50 to 55 minutes, or until a toothpick inserted in the center of the custard comes out clean. Allow to cool for 20 to 30 minutes.

Meanwhile, make the crumble. In a food processor, combine the walnuts, dates, cinnamon, and salt and blend until the nuts are chopped and the ingredients are well combined. Top each ramekin with some of the crumble and serve.

EGG-FREE VERSION

This custard can be made egg-free by first combining 2 tablespoons chia seeds with 6 tablespoons warm water. Let the mixture sit for 15 minutes, then whisk with a fork before stirring into the other custard ingredients in place of the eggs. Note that the custard won't firm up as readily in the oven as a result, but cooling it in the refrigerator for 3 to 4 hours after baking will produce the desired texture.

Sinfully Silky Chocolate Mousse

I changed the name of this recipe from "sane and silky" to "sinfully silky" because who wants to think about being sane when eating dessert? But the truth is, there's nothing sinful about this dessert. I realize you might be skeptical when you see tofu and avocado in the ingredient list, but trust me, you'll be rewarded with a light, smooth, chocolaty treat that will help you tame the sugar beast. The almond extract is optional but definitely gives this treat more of an Almond Joy quality. You can even top it with some unsweetened shredded coconut to complete the picture.

Makes 4 servings

10 ounces silken tofu
1 small or ½ large avocado
½ cup unsweetened cocoa powder

⅓ cup agave nectar or pure
  maple syrup
1 teaspoon almond extract (optional)

In a blender or food processor, blend all the ingredients until silky smooth. Taste and add more sweetener, 1 teaspoon at a time, if necessary. Transfer the mousse into dessert glasses, cover, and chill in the refrigerator for a few hours or overnight for the best texture.

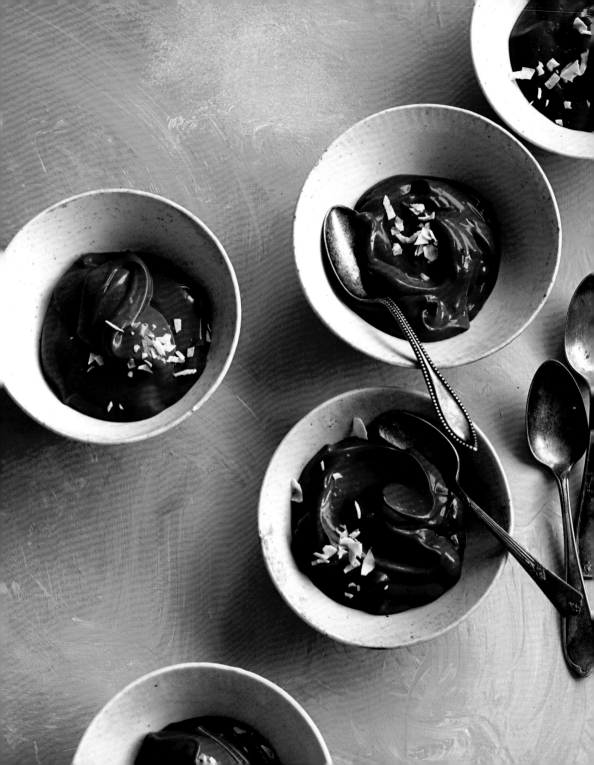

Coconut-Lime Bites

Any dessert that features avocados and walnuts is a nutritional winner in my book. If you associate avocados only with guacamole and savory dishes, you'll be pleasantly surprised at how well they perform in a creamy, dreamy dessert. I initially made this as a pie, which might be a bit less labor intensive if you don't want to fuss with the muffin cups. But I love having these as a single-serving mini treat. I'd like to say it's built-in portion control, but sometimes it's hard to eat just one. Note that the coconut milk needs to be refrigerated overnight.

Makes 2 dozen bites

3 cups walnuts
10 Medjool dates, pitted
¼ teaspoon sea salt
1 vanilla bean
2 medium avocados, halved
¾ cup freshly squeezed lime juice

½ teaspoon freshly grated lime zest
⅓ cup agave nectar or raw honey
1 tablespoon coconut flour
2 (14-ounce) cans full-fat, unsweet-
    ened coconut milk, refrigerated
    overnight

In a food processor, combine the walnuts, dates, and salt. Use a paring knife to slice the vanilla bean lengthwise down the center. Open the bean to expose the paste-like seeds, use the back of the knife to gently scrape them out of the pod, and add them to the food processor. Blend the ingredients until finely chopped and well combined.

In a 24-cup nonstick mini-muffin tin, press a thin layer of the walnut mixture into the bottoms and sides of each cup (as you would a piecrust). Set aside.

Place a medium (preferably metal) mixing bowl in the freezer for 10 minutes. Scoop the avocados into the clean food processor. Add the lime juice and zest, agave, and flour. Blend until smooth and creamy.

Remove the coconut milk from the refrigerator without shaking the cans. Scoop out the hardened coconut cream from both cans and place in the chilled mixing bowl. (To avoid getting the liquid coconut milk, try opening the can upside down, pouring off the liquid first, then scooping out the cream.) Reserve the liquid coconut milk for another use (it can be a great addition to smoothies!). Using a hand mixer, whip the coconut cream until it's fluffy and resembles true whipped cream, which can take 3 to 5 minutes. Fold the avocado mixture into the whipped cream and stir until well combined.

Carefully pour the cream mixture into the walnut crusts, filling each cup to the top. Place the tin in the freezer for 2 to 3 hours, then allow the bites to thaw slightly before serving. Store any extras in the refrigerator or freezer.

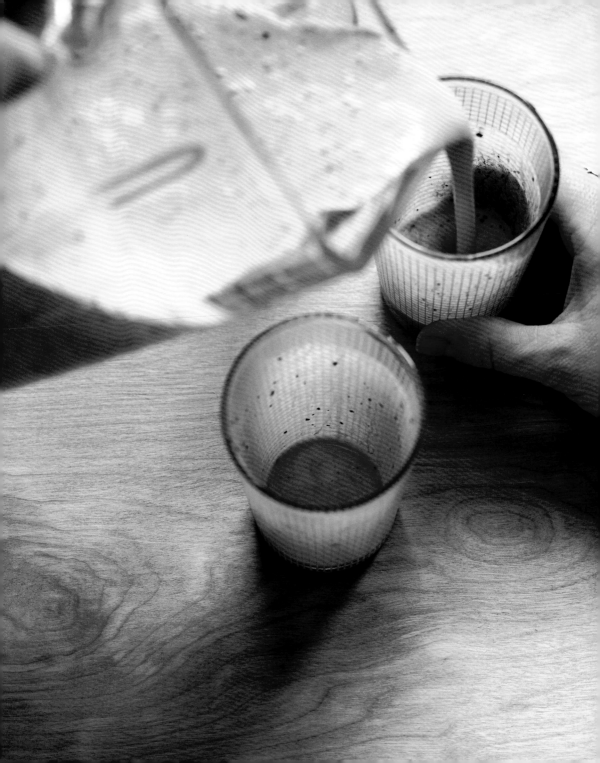

Acknowledgments

»»««

This book was definitely a labor of love and an attempt to broaden my reach so that more people can learn how to benefit from the healing powers of food. I was somewhat awestruck by the feedback I got from my last book, *Anti-Inflammatory Eating Made Easy*, and I am so grateful for the people who found their way to my book and shared their success stories with me. I have to thank Gary Luke, CEO and publisher at Sasquatch Books, who encouraged me to write that book and then immediately asked, "What's next?"

I've had a lot of people in my life affected by depression and anxiety, so this topic is close to my heart. I give credit to Dr. James Gordon, founder and executive director of the Center for Mind-Body Medicine (CMBM), who wrote the brilliant book *Unstuck: Your Guide to the Seven-Stage Journey Out of Depression*. That book highlighted the effectiveness of a holistic treatment plan for depression and showcased the relevance of nutrition. It motivated me to take the professional training course through CMBM and I use those principles with my patients in my private practice every day.

My work as a nutritionist, author, and cooking instructor is so rewarding and I can't imagine doing anything else. I doubt I ever would have had the courage to leave my career in public relations and head back to school to become a dietitian had it not been for Barb Schiltz, my dear friend and mentor. She gave me a swift kick in the pants and told me take the leap. My education at Bastyr University just confirmed that I was on the right path, and I was fortunate enough to have inspiring teachers like Kelly Morrow, Cynthia Lair, and Debra Boutin. Their dedication to the field is nothing short of extraordinary.

And then there are the foodies in my life who share my passion for interesting, creative, healthy, delicious food. We love to read about it, talk about it, and write it about, and we take great pleasure in sharing meals together.

Barb Schiltz, Katherine Oldfield, Greg Janssen, Heather King, Deanna Minich, and Maribeth Evezich—you are my people!

I like to focus on the *art* of cooking, but developing recipes and writing a cookbook is more of a *science* and requires some precision and lots of instructions. My trusted recipe testers take their jobs very seriously, giving me thoughtful feedback and invaluable input that make each recipe more delicious and easier to follow. A *huge* thank-you to Gabrielle Avina, Bill Babb, Kim Campbell, Amy Ecklund, Lisa Miller, Reis Pearson, Karen Pfeiffer Bush, Katie Quinn, Rob and Julie Sweet, and Tina Watson. This book is better because of you.

Bibliography

>>»«<

Appleton, K. M., P. J. Rogers, and A. R. Ness. "Updated Systematic Review and Meta-Analysis of the Effects of n−3 Long-Chain Polyunsaturated Fatty Acids on Depressed Mood." *American Journal of Clinical Nutrition* 91, no. 3 (March 2010): 757–770.

Bertone-Johnson, E. R., S. I. Powers, L. Spangler, R. L. Brunner, Y. L. Michael, J. C. Larson, A. E. Millen, M. N. Bueche, E. Salmoirago-Blotcher, S. Liu, S. Wassertheil-Smoller, J. K. Ockene, I. Ockene, and J. E. Manson. "Vitamin D Intake from Foods and Supplements and Depressive Symptoms in a Diverse Population of Older Women." *American Journal of Clinical Nutrition* 94, no. 4 (October 2011): 1104–12.

Bested, A. C., A. C. Logan, and E. M. Selhub. "Intestinal Microbiota, Probiotics and Mental Health: From Metchnikoff to Modern Advances. Part III – Convergence Toward Clinical Trials." *Gut Pathogens* 5, no. 4 (March 2013).

Bielland, I., G. S. Tell, and S. E. Vollset. "Choline in Anxiety and Depression: The Hordaland Health Study." *American Journal of Clinical Nutrition* 90, no. 4 (October 2009): 1056–1060.

Grosso, G., A. Pajak, and S. Marventano. "Role of Omega-3 Fatty Acids in the Treatment of Depressive Disorders: A Comprehensive Meta-Analysis of Randomized Clinical Trials." *PLoS ONE* 9, no. 5 (2014): e96905.

Hibbeln, J. "Fish Consumption and Major Depression." *The Lancet* 351, no. 9110 (April 1998): 1213.

Jacka, F. N., and N. Cherbuin. "Dietary Patterns and Depressive Symptoms over Time: Examining the Relationships with Socioeconomic Position, Health Behaviors and Cardiovascular Risk." *PLoS ONE* 9, no. 1 (2014): e87657. doi: 10.1371.

Logan, A. C. "Omega-3 Fatty Acids and Major Depression: A Primer for the Mental Health Professional." *Lipids in Health and Disease* 3, no. 25 (2004).

Mayer, E. A. "Gut Feelings: The Emerging Biology of Gut-Brain Communication." *Nature Reviews Neuroscience* 12, no. 8 (July 2013).

Molteni, R., and R. J. Barnard. "A High-Fat, Refined Sugar Diet Reduces Hippocampal Brain-Derived Neurotrophic Factor, Neuronal Plasticity, and Learning." *Neuroscience* 112, no. 4 (July 2002): 803–14.

Naleid, A. M., J. W. Grimm, and D. A. Kessler. "Deconstructing the Vanilla Milkshake: The Dominant Effect of Sucrose on Self-Administration of Nutrient-Flavor Mixtures." *Appetite* 50, no. 1 (January 2008): 128–38.

Niu, K., H. Guo, and M. Kakizaki. "A Tomato-Rich Diet is Related to Depressive Symptoms among an Elderly Population Aged 70 Years and Over: A Population-Based, Cross-Sectional Analysis." *Journal of Affective Disorders* 144, no. 1-2 (January 2013): 165–70.

Patrick, R. P., and B. N. Ames. "Vitamin D Hormone Regulates Serotonin Synthesis. Part 1: Relevance for Autism." *The FASEB Journal* 28, no. 6 (February 2014): 2398–2413.

Peet, M. "International Variations in the Outcome of Schizophrenia and the Prevalence of Depression in Relation to National Dietary Practices: An Ecological Analysis." *British Journal of Psychiatry* 184, no. 5 (May 2004): 404–8.

Sánchez-Villegas, A., and E. Toledo. "Fast-Food and Commercial Baked Goods Consumption and the Risk of Depression." *Public Health Nutrition* 15, no. 3 (March 2012): 424–32.

Sánchez-Villegas, A., and M. Delgado-Rodriguez. "Association of the Mediterranean Dietary Pattern with the Incidence of Depression." *Archives of General Psychiatry* 66, no. 10 (October 2009): 1090–1098.

Sarris, J., and A. Logan. "Nutritional Medicine as Mainstream in Psychiatry." *The Lancet Psychiatry* 2, no. 3 (March 2015): 271–274.

Spedding, S. "Vitamin D and Depression: A Systematic Review and Meta-Analysis Comparing Studies with and without Biological Flaws." *Nutrients* 6, no. 4 (April 2014): 1501–1518.

Stice, E., and S. Spoor. "Relation Between Obesity and Blunted Striatal Response to Food Is Moderated by TaqIA A1 Allele." *Science* 322, no. 5900 (October 2008): 449–52.

Vargas, H. O., and S. O. Nunes. "Oxidative Stress and Lowered Total Antioxidant Status Are Associated with a History of Suicide Attempts." *Journal of Affective Disorders* 150, no. 3 (September 2013): 923–30.

Wansink, B., M. M. Cheney, and N. Chan. "Exploring Comfort Food Preferences across Gender and Age." *Physiology and Behavior* 79, no. 4-5 (September 2003): 739–747.

Yannakoulia, M., D. B. Panagiotakos, and C. Pitsavos. "Eating Habits in Relations to Anxiety Symptoms among Apparently Healthy Adults. A Pattern Analysis from the ATTICA Study." *Appetite* 51, no. 3 (November 2008): 519–25.

Index

>> >> << <<

squash and zucchini
Delicata Squash with Quinoa-Pecan
Stuffing, *100*, 101
Spaghetti Squash Carbonara with
Sautéed Vegetables, 98–99
Zoodles Marinara with Turkey Meat-
balls, *88*, 89–90
Standard American Diet (SAD), 1–2, 17
sugar addiction, overcoming, 7–8
Sunchoke and Celeriac Soup, Silky,
121, 122

T

Thai Peanut Bowl, Spicy, 105
tofu
Sinfully Silky Chocolate Mousse,
160, *161*
soy, health benefits of, 72, 96
Spicy Tahini Tofu Bites, 72
Tofu Breakfast Scramble, 51
Tofu Taco Salad, 96, *97*
Torte, Chocolate Pear, 155–156, *157*
Tortilla Soup with Black Beans,
Spicy, 120

W

walnuts
Coconut-Lime Bites, 162–163
health benefits of, 61
Honey-Glazed Walnuts with
Cinnamon Spice, 61

Y

Yam and Brussels Sprout Hash with
Smoked Salmon, 54
Yam and Kale Salad, Smoky, 116
Yams and Green Eggs, 52
Yogurt, Soy, 143
Yogurt Swirl, Raspberry, *146*, 147

Z

zucchini. *See* squash and zucchini

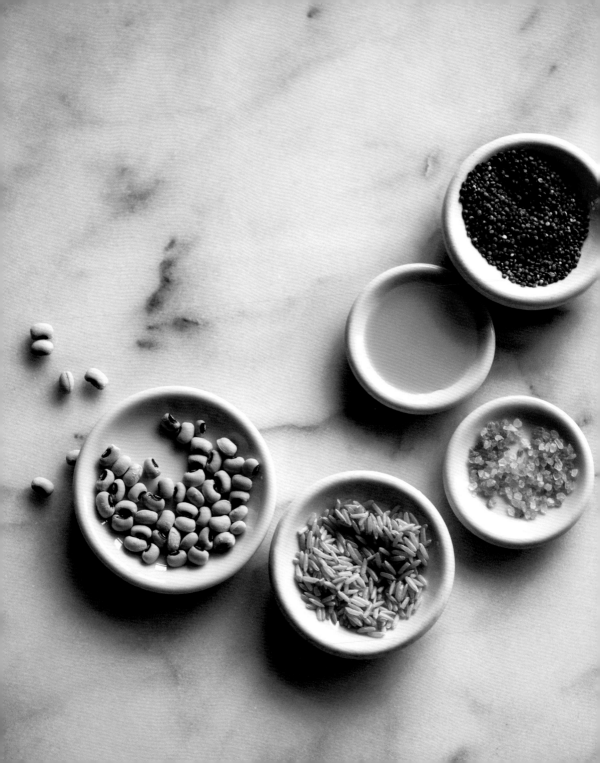

Conversions

VOLUME

US	METRIC	IMPERIAL
¼ tsp.	1.25 ml	
½ tsp.	2.5 ml	
1 tsp.	5 ml	
½ Tbsp.	7.5 ml	
1 Tbsp.	15 ml	
⅛ c.	30 ml	1 fl. oz.
¼ c.	60 ml	2 fl. oz.
⅓ c.	80 ml	2.5 fl. oz.
½ c.	125 ml	4 fl. oz.
1 c.	250 ml	8 fl. oz.
2 c. (1 pt.)	500 ml	16 fl. oz.
1 qt.	1 l	32 fl. oz.

LENGTH

US	METRIC
⅛ in.	3 mm
¼ in.	6 mm
½ in.	1.25 cm
1 in.	2.5 cm
1 ft.	30 cm

WEIGHT

AVOIRDUPOIS	METRIC
¼ oz.	7 g
½ oz.	15 g
1 oz.	30 g
2 oz.	60 g
3 oz.	90 g
4 oz.	115 g
5 oz.	150 g
6 oz.	175 g
7 oz.	200 g
8 oz. (½ lb.)	225 g
9 oz.	250 g
10 oz.	300 g
11 oz.	325 g
12 oz.	350 g
13 oz.	375 g
14 oz.	400 g
15 oz.	425 g
16 oz. (1 lb.)	450 g
1½ lb.	750 g
2 lb.	900 g
2¼ lb.	1 kg
3 lb.	1.4 kg
4 lb.	1.8 kg

TEMPERATURE

OVEN MARK	FAHRENHEIT	CELSIUS	GAS
Very cool	250–275	130–140	½–1
Cool	300	150	2
Warm	325	165	3
Moderate	350	175	4
Moderately hot	375	190	5
	400	200	6
Hot	425	220	7
	450	230	8
Very Hot	475	245	9

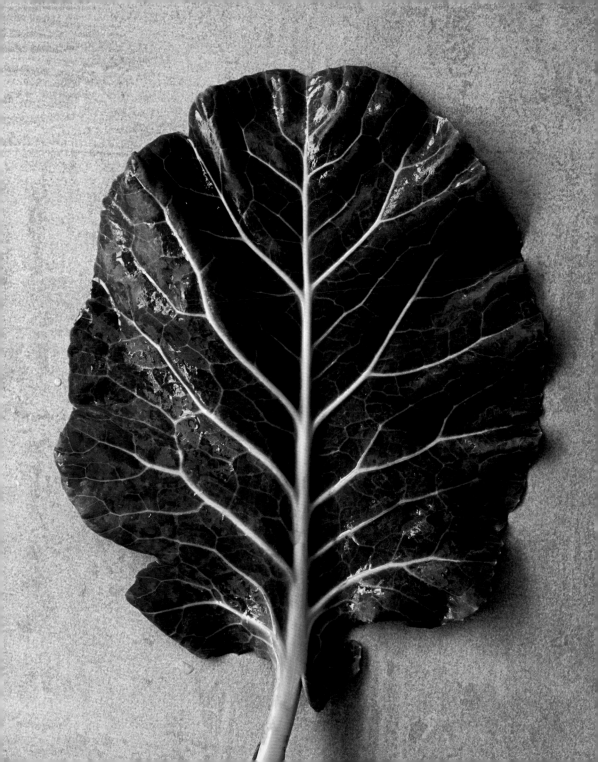

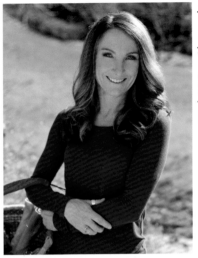

Nicole M. Ryan Photography

About the Author

»»««

MICHELLE BABB is a registered dietitian with a private practice in West Seattle, where she specializes in mind-body nutrition, weight management, and inflammatory digestive disorders.

Michelle developed a passion for cooking when she was a student at Bastyr, and now teaches nutrition-focused cooking classes at Puget Consumers Co-op. Her recipes often feature underappreciated ingredients, like beets, brussels sprouts, and sunchokes. She takes great pleasure in converting dubious meat and potato lovers into vegetable enthusiasts.

When she's not in the kitchen, Michelle enjoys running, kayaking, sailing, and traveling. She also loves to write and is the author of *Anti-Inflammatory Eating Made Easy* and coauthor of *The Imperfect Perfectionist: Seasonal Secrets for a Happy and Balanced Life*. Learn more about Michelle at EatPlayBe.com.

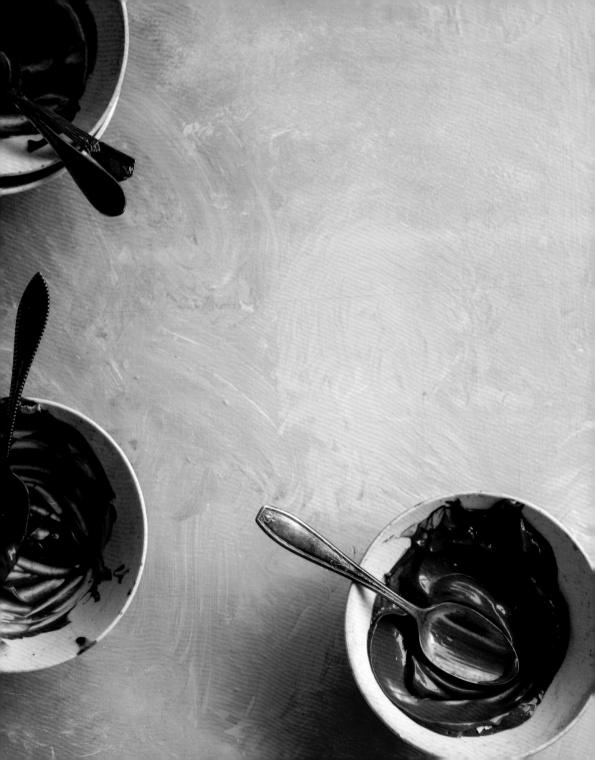